Surgical Talk

Lecture Notes in Undergraduate Surgery

3rd Edition

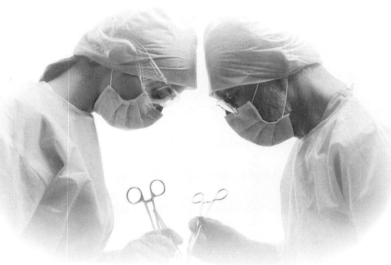

Andrew Goldberg

The Royal National Orthopaedic Hospital Trust, Stanmore, UK &
University College London, UK

Gerard Stansby

Newcastle University & Freeman Hospital,
Newcastle upon Tyne, UK

 Imperial College Press

Published by

Imperial College Press
57 Shelton Street
Covent Garden
London WC2H 9HE

Distributed by

World Scientific Publishing Co. Pte. Ltd.
5 Toh Tuck Link, Singapore 596224
USA office: 27 Warren Street, Suite 401-402, Hackensack, NJ 07601
UK office: 57 Shelton Street, Covent Garden, London WC2H 9HE

British Library Cataloguing-in-Publication Data
A catalogue record for this book is available from the British Library.

SURGICAL TALK
Lecture Notes in Undergraduate Surgery
(3rd Edition)

ISBN-13 978-1-84816-614-1 (pbk)
ISBN-10 1-84816-614-1 (pbk)

Typeset by Stallion Press
Email: enquiries@stallionpress.com

Printed by FuIsland Offset Printing (S) Pte Ltd Singapore

LIVER/PANC
OES/STOMACH
SM INT + COLON X X
Rectum + Anus
Acute abdo
BREAST
(HERNIAS)
Vasc
Urology
Ov thg

CONTE

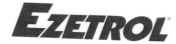

CONTRIBUTORS

Mr Ben Bannerjee MD, FRCS.
Consultant Surgeon and Honorary Senior Lecturer,
Sunderland Royal Hospitals, Sunderland, UK.

Mr Richard M Charnley DM, FRCS.
Consultant Hepato-pancreato-biliary Surgeon,
Freeman Hospital, Newcastle upon Tyne, UK.

Mr Jeremy French MD FRCS.
Consultant Hepato-pancreato-biliary Surgeon,
Freeman Hospital, Newcastle upon Tyne, UK.

Mr Jonathan Glass FRCS (Urol).
Consultant Urologist, Guy's and St Thomas' Hospital NHS Trust,
London, UK.

Prof. S Michael Griffin MD, FRCS.
Professor of Gastrointestinal Surgery,
Northern Oesophagogastric Unit, Royal Victoria Infirmary,
Newcastle upon Tyne, UK.

Ms Monica Hansrani MD, FRCS.
Consultant Vascular Surgeon, James Cook University Hospital,
Middlesbrough, UK.

Mr Alan F Horgan MD, FRCS.
Consultant Colorectal Surgeon, Freeman Hospital,
Newcastle upon Tyne, UK.

Prof. Tom Lennard MD, FRCS.
Professor of Breast and Endocrine Surgery, Royal Victoria Infirmary
Newcastle University, UK.

Mr Ashraf Morgan MS, FRCSI.
Senior Specialist ENT, Pilgrim Hospital,
Boston, Lincolnshire, UK.

Dr Ian Nesbitt FRCA, Dip ICM.
Consultant Anaesthetist, Freeman Hospital,
Newcastle upon Tyne, UK.

Mr Michael Oko FRCS.
Consultant ENT Surgeon, Pilgrim Hospital,
Boston, Lincolnshire, UK.

Ms Sarah Robinson FRCS.
Research Registrar, Northern Oesophagogastric Unit,
Royal Victoria Infirmary, Newcastle upon Tyne, UK.

Mr Peter Smitham PhD, FRCS.
Clinical Lecturer, Royal National Orthopaedic Hospital NHS Trust,
Stanmore, UK.

Mr Philip D Yates FRCS.
Consultant ENT Surgeon, Freeman Hospital,
Newcastle upon Tyne, UK.

FOREWORD TO THE FIRST EDITION

The authors are to be congratulated on a clearly written and presented text. Using this book, the student can build up a firm foundation of both knowledge and skills, which will not only enable the hurdle of finals to be negotiated with confidence, but will also be of everyday value in clinical practice.

Visually attractive, readable and scientifically sound, the book makes relatively light work of the large volume of information contained within.

It seems likely to me that this book will appeal not only to students with final examinations in mind, but also to house surgeons and senior house officers with patients to diagnose and treat and, perhaps, with the MRCS on the horizon.

Professor Averil Mansfield CBE, ChM, FRCS

PREFACE TO THE FIRST EDITION

When you are a medical student, finals seem a daunting prospect. However, the truth is that most candidates pass the exam easily and most junior doctors look back at finals as being relatively straightforward. The reason for this is that this exam is simply the last hurdle in a long and draining race and by the time you have reached this point, the odds are with you to finish the course. The examiners are not there to fail candidates *per se*; in fact, the opposite is true and they are really trying to help you pass. However, they must ensure that a safe junior doctor is unleashed on the public. Because of this fact you must know the basics of all the common emergency situations. Luck plays only a small part in finals for most students and, as someone once said, "The harder you work, the luckier you get."

The philosophy of this book is to focus on the level of knowledge and the approach that would be expected of the better students arriving at finals. We have tried to include as much as possible without making the book too cumbersome. No book of this scope can include every possible topic, but we hope that we have included all that could legitimately be expected of you for the final exam. The book also contains comprehensive sections on trauma, orthopaedics and urology, which so often get left out of other texts, and a section on fluid balance that may continue to be of use when you are a junior house officer.

The text has been deliberately written in a tutorial-like story format as opposed to a set of lists, since this makes it easier to understand and remember. Everyone loves a list but we must assure you that you are much more likely to remember a list if you have written it yourself. Therefore, space has been left adjacent to the text for you to pick out important details from the text and jot down your own lists. If you do this as you go along, you will effectively produce your own textbook which will become an invaluable tool, with all you need for success at your fingertips.

Good luck with your revision and the exam, and we hope this book will help.

Andy Goldberg
Gerry Stansby

PREFACE TO THE SECOND EDITION

We were delighted with the positive feedback that the first edition received from medical students as well as many junior doctors who had long passed their final examinations yet still found the book useful in their working lives.

Over the last few years, the world of medicine has moved on with advances in almost every field. With this in mind, we decided to bring the text up to date and to bring in experts to co-author many of the chapters, especially those in which we were no longer experts! Each chapter has been reviewed and updated by the co-author whose name is listed at the beginning of each chapter. In addition, we have added an entirely new chapter on ENT, making *Surgical Talk* one of the only texts which comprehensively reviews all of the surgical specialities required for final surgical examinations.

We hope that those of you at that scary point in your career, namely just before you start a job in a new specialty, will also find this book a great overview of the subjects you need to know.

The teaching focus of the text remains. It is still full of "top tips" to keep the reader one step ahead of the examiner. Exams are a mechanism to sell books. So consider this book a mechanism to pass exams. All feedback is welcome and we look forward to hearing from you.

Andy Goldberg
Gerry Stansby

PREFACE TO THE THIRD EDITION

It is now ten years since the first edition was published and we were delighted to be asked to produce a third edition of the text to bring it up to date.

We started this journey to fulfil demands from medical students, and our passion for helping students to get up to speed remains as strong.

Now, as we are armed with a few more grey hairs, it is reassuring to occasionally meet a fellow consultant who used the original book to pass their exams and to hear a note of gratitude from them.

One of the main pieces of feedback we received about previous editions was that it looked anything but stimulating on the bookshelf! Students often commented that if it wasn't for word of mouth they would have never given the book a second look. They are always pleased that they did. We are therefore delighted that the publishers have agreed to revise all of the images and diagrams for the third edition; with the addition of colour, we hope that it will also appeal to those who don't just rely on personal recommendation.

We remain proud that this is the only textbook out there that contains comprehensive chapters on ENT, orthopaedics and urology, as well as detailed sections on things like fluid balance, rarely found in other undergraduate texts. This means that you don't have to buy endless revision aids to ensure you have all the topics covered.

To accompany this book we have also written a revision guide, composed of hundreds of MCQs and EMQs for surgical finals, entitled *Surgery: Problems and Solutions. Revision Questions in Undergraduate Surgery*. The texts are synergistic and hopefully provide a mechanism for you to learn your subjects and then challenge yourself with mock exams.

Once more, good luck with your learning and with any exams. We hope this book will help you to prepare and develop your confidence for the challenges that lie ahead.

All feedback is welcome and we look forward to hearing from you.

Andy Goldberg
Gerry Stansby

ABOUT THE EDITORS

Mr Andy Goldberg MBBS, MD, FRCS (Tr&Orth)

Andy Goldberg qualified from the Imperial College School of Medicine in 1994. His specialist training was in trauma and orthopaedics on the North East Thames Programme. In April 2010 he was appointed to his current role as Clinical Senior Lecturer in Trauma and Orthopaedics at UCL, Institute of Orthopaedics and Musculoskeletal Science, and an Honorary Consultant Orthopaedic Surgeon at the Royal National Orthopaedic Hospital NHS Trust, in Stanmore, UK. He is a fellow of the Royal College of Surgeons of England and Ireland and a member of the British Orthopaedic Association, the British Orthopaedic Foot & Ankle Society and the Orthopaedic Research Society. He has an MD thesis on cartilage repair, based on pioneering work using human mesenchymal stem cells, awarded by the University of London in 2006. Andy sits on a number of company boards and committees and runs several master's level student courses at UCL. He founded the Medical Futures Innovation Awards in 2001, which has since become one of the UK's highest healthcare accolades and assists medical professionals in developing their innovative ideas. He was honoured with an OBE in the Queen's New Year's Honours List 2011 for services to medicine.

Professor Gerry Stansby MA (Cantab), MB, MChir, FRCS

Gerry Stansby qualified from Cambridge University and Addenbrooke's Hospital in 1982. In 1993, he went to St Mary's Hospital in London as a Senior Clinical Vascular Fellow and, in 1994, became Senior Lecturer in General and Vascular Surgery at St Mary's Hospital and Imperial College,

London. In January 2000, he obtained his current position of Professor of Vascular Surgery at the University of Newcastle and the Freeman Hospital. He is the author of more than 200 scientific articles and several books. He is a coordinating editor for the Cochrane Peripheral Vascular Diseases Group and several medical journals. He is Chair of the North of England Cardiovascular network group for vascular surgery and Director of the North East aneurysm screening project. He is a regular examiner at medical finals both in the UK and overseas.

ACKNOWLEDGEMENTS

To our *parents* and *wives* who are always there for us and always a forethought. To our amazing *children* who give us reason to teach, share knowledge and enjoy what we do.

To all the *contributing authors* who brought their invaluable depth of expertise. To all of the *medical students*, for their suggestions before and after the books in this series were written.

1

SURGICAL TALK

Andy Goldberg and Gerry Stansby

There is no doubt that the best performers in finals are those candidates who think logically, express themselves clearly and avoid putting their foot in their mouth by saying something stupid. Their depth of knowledge is not necessarily greater than that of their fellow candidates, but they do well in every part of the exam — written, clinical and viva.

The message is clear: you must start early, practising a systematic approach to the subject. In this chapter several examples of such approaches are given. You may not like all of them, so choose a method that suits you and spend a great deal of time perfecting it. Also note that a short pause before answering does not detract from the answer and may avoid a dreadful mistake.

Remember also that in finals the examiners are looking for a minimum standard across the breadth of medicine and surgery. Effectively, they wish to assess whether you will be safe as a junior doctor subsequently. They will not be impressed by superb knowledge in one area if there is ignorance about basic facts in another. You will not be expected to know the technical details of any particular operation but you should have an understanding of the broad principles and common complications that would have to be explained to the patient. An example question might be "What would you warn this patient about when obtaining consent from them for this operation?" If you do not know that there is a risk of dying or that there is a high chance of needing a colostomy, then how could you be expected to have any meaningful dialogue with the patient or to build their trust?

It follows that it is in your best interest to make sure that you know the essential basics about all relevant topics before attempting to learn some topics in greater detail. It is also a basic fact of human psychology that, when revising, students tend to revise more often the areas they feel comfortable with. In fact it is the areas you feel uncomfortable with that you need to spend time on! To avoid leaving gaps in your revision, take the chapter headings of your surgical textbook and make sure that you feel you can give a short summary of the basic points in each chapter. If you cannot say much about a particular subject (and would dread being asked about it in the finals), then that is your most urgent revision priority — do not leave it to chance.

SURGICAL SIEVES

Sometimes you are asked an obscure question, which throws you off. Your mind goes blank, you blurt out the first thing that comes into your head and you end up in a deep hole. Often you realise afterwards that you did know the answer, or at least some of it. A sieve allows you to gather your thoughts, working from first principles, and come up with at least some sensible statements. When you answer a question you should really talk about the most common things first and the rarities at the end, and one disadvantage of using a sieve is that you may not be able to rapidly reorganise your thoughts in this way. Still, it is useful when all else fails and it is invaluable in essay writing.

The Aetiological Sieve

- Congenital
- Acquired
  - Traumatic
  - Inflammatory (physical, chemical, infective)
  - Neoplastic (benign or malignant, primary or secondary)
  - Circulatory
  - Autoimmune
  - Nutritional
  - Metabolic

o Endocrine
o Drugs
o Degenerative
o Iatrogenic
o Psychosomatic

TIN CAN MED DIP is one way of remembering it, but you probably have your own method.

The Anatomical Sieve

The anatomical sieve can apply to anatomical sites, structures or tissue types. If asked "What are the causes of mechanical bowel obstruction?", you could say "Adhesions". This is a correct answer but not an ideal way of saying it.

Another approach might be to start by saying that the bowel is a structure consisting of several anatomical regions and hence obstruction can occur anywhere along its length; for example, stomach outflow obstruction, small bowel obstruction and large bowel obstruction. The examiner will then usually pick one route and lead you along it. If writing an answer you would of course need to discuss all three.

Then you could add that the bowel is a hollow tube, and like any hollow tube (cf. ureters) it can become blocked at three sites: from outside the tube pressing in (extramural), within the wall of the tube (intramural) and within the lumen of the tube (luminal). Where appropriate, answers could then be structured as shown in Table 1.1.

Do not forget that there are other structures such as muscles, bones, joints and nerves in the region, but in this case these would rarely be the

Table 1.1. Causes of Mechanical Bowel Obstruction

Extramural	Intramural	Luminal
Adhesions	Inflammation (e.g. Crohn's)	Impacted faeces
Strangulated hernia	Tumours	Large polyps
Extrinsic compression	Infarction	Foreign body
Volvulus	Strictures	Intussusception

cause. If possible, when listing differential diagnoses, try to do so in the order of their likelihood (i.e. do not mention vanishingly rare things before common things).

General and Specific

"Tell me about postoperative complications." When asked such a question it is difficult to know where to start. As before, you must avoid saying the first thing that comes into your head, as this may not be the most relevant. Here, an approach is to use two types of classification: one by type of complication and the other by time scale.

Postoperative complications can be general, i.e. applying to any operation (such as the effects of anaesthesia), or specific, i.e. applying to a particular operation (such as damage to the recurrent laryngeal nerve in thyroidectomy).

Once classified into general and specific complications, they can be broken down further by time scale. These complications can be immediate, early or late (see the chapter on pre- and postoperative complications for further examples).

Once you use these principles, it becomes easy to answer most questions logically. For example: "What are the causes of haematuria?" The causes can be general (e.g. a bleeding disorder or use of anticoagulants) or specific, relating to any of the anatomical structures in the region. Table 1.2 shows the possible causes relating to the structures (starting from the top) that are part of the urinary tract.

In this example, don't forget to confirm true haematuria, since the appearance of red urine can occur following beetroot ingestion or the use

Table 1.2.   Specific Causes of Haematuria

Structure	Causes
Kidney	Stones, trauma, carcinoma (use the aetiological sieve)
Ureter	Tumour, stones, infection
Bladder	Infection, tumour, stones
Prostate	Benign hypertrophy, tumour, infection
Urethra	Stones, infection, trauma

of certain drugs such as rifampicin. Also exclude bleeding from the vagina or anus.

Tissue Type

Try to take a few minutes to list the possible causes of a lump in the groin. It's quite hard to do so, and you may find it difficult to be exhaustive. A good method to use here is classification by tissue type. So, for example, you would say, "A lump can arise from any of the tissue types in this region." Table 1.3 gives some examples.

Investigations

Imagine being asked "How would you investigate such a patient?" It would be easy to shout out "Full blood count", "Chest X-ray" or "Calcium" as an answer. It's much more difficult to be systematic and methodical. We recommend that you break down investigations in the following manner:

- Simple urine and faecal tests (e.g. urine dipstick, microscopy and culture, pregnancy tests, faecal occult blood)
- Haematological tests (routine, e.g. full blood count; or special, e.g. tumour markers)
- Radiological tests (e.g. chest X-ray, ultrasound or CT)
- Special investigations (e.g. gastroscopy, V/Q scans)

Table 1.3. Possible Causes of a Lump in the Groin Classified by Tissue Type

Tissue type	Example
Skin	Sebaceous cyst
Adipose tissue	Lipoma
Connective tissue	Fibroma
Lymphatics	Enlarged lymph node
Blood vessels	Saphena varix, femoral artery aneurysm
Inguinal canal	Inguinal hernia, hydrocoele of the cord
Femoral canal	Femoral hernia
Testes	Undescended testes

You may be asked to justify your choice of investigation. Often we send off investigations as a baseline since the patients are being admitted to hospital. This is justified in the elderly but is usually a waste of resources in young, fit patients. A full blood count is justified in young females, to check for anaemia. Urea and electrolytes (U&E) should be sent for patients on diuretics.

Management

"Discuss the treatment of benign prostatic hypertrophy" is a different question from "Discuss the management of benign prostatic hypertrophy". In the former the examiners want you to purely concentrate on treatment and not on diagnosis. In your answer you should define benign prostatic hypertrophy and perhaps say one or two sentences on the condition and its investigation, but do not spend too long on this as you will get no extra marks. A discussion of its management involves discussing all of the steps that deal with the clinical problem, including the history, examination, investigations, formation of a diagnosis and treatment.

When discussing treatment you can again break down your answer into subheadings. For example, treatment can be conservative, medical or surgical. In this case, the answer can be broken down as follows:

- *Conservative*. This usually means ruling out cancer. A prostate-specific antigen (PSA) of less than 4 and a normal examination would help the doctor to be comfortable about reassuring the patient to follow a policy of watchful waiting unless the symptoms get worse.
- *Medical*. For example, drugs such as α_1-adrenoreceptor blockers or 5-α-reductase inhibitors.
- *Surgical*. For example, transurethral resection of the prostate (TURP).

Answering an Essay

Many medical schools have stopped setting essays. If you are asked to write an essay, note that the questions might be quite general; for example, "Minimal access surgery — discuss". The following is a guide for the headings you can use in writing such an essay; some surgeons refer to this as the pathological sieve.

- Definition
- Aetiology (incidence, age, sex, geography) and risk factors
- Histology (macro and micro)
- Clinical features (signs and symptoms)
- Diagnosis (and differential diagnosis)
- Clinical staging (if appropriate)
- Investigations/treatment/management
- Complications
- Prognosis

Remember that management depends on diagnosis and that diagnosis depends on the history, examination and special investigations. Therefore, management refers to all of the steps of clinical assessment and investigation as well as treatment.

Never forget the steps of management which occur early on as the patient is being admitted to hospital. For example, if asked how you would manage a case of acute cholecystitis, you need to say that you would give the patient adequate analgesia, arrange admission to a surgical bed, put up a drip, keep the patient nil by mouth, etc., before talking about liver function tests or ultrasound scans (which would not normally be available immediately). It is often a good idea to try to imagine that you are actually the doctor in A&E who is trying to sort the patient out. What would you actually do? What observations would you ask the nurses to take? When would you review the patient? Would you inform someone more senior? Would you put in a urinary catheter? By mentioning such points you not only increase the content of your answer, you also demonstrate that you have become aware of the practical aspects of being a junior doctor as well as of the textbook theory.

As part of your discussion of management it is worth considering adding the acronym "POSSET" at the end of an essay if appropriate. It stands for Physio, Occupational therapy, Specialists (e.g. stoma care nurse, breast care nurse, speech therapists, etc.), Social workers,

Education and Terminal care. The last two are of the utmost importance. Education involves explaining things like when the stitches will come out, what the patient can and cannot do (such as when the patient can drive, have sex, etc.). Terminal care means involving the Macmillan nurses, arranging for the syringe pump to deliver analgesia, speaking to the GP, etc. This last paragraph can be the difference between a good essay and an excellent one.

History of a Lump

Surgery is full of lumps. No matter where the lump is, there are only five questions you need to remember when taking the history of a lump:

- When and how did you first notice the lump?
- How has the lump changed since you first noticed it?
- What symptoms does it cause you?
- Have you got any more or have you had this before?
- What do you think it is?

You must learn this list. These are the vital questions and they apply to any lump, whether it is in the neck, in the breast or in the groin. We now explore these questions in more detail.

- *When and how did you first notice the lump?* Was it noticed incidentally, whilst looking in the mirror, or did the patient's partner point it out? Remember that this asks when the lump was first noticed and not when it first appeared.
- *How has the lump changed?* Has it got bigger, smaller, stayed the same size or has it come and gone? Has it changed its appearance and consistency, does it get bigger during a menstrual period?
- *What symptoms does it cause you?* Is it painful? (Patients often wrongly equate this to cancer.) Symptoms usually are related to anatomical site. For example, in breast lumps, is there nipple discharge? A lump in the neck could affect voice, respiration or eating. If you think this is a thyroid lump, ask relevant questions about the symptoms of hypo- or hyperthyroidism.

- *Have you got any more/had it before?* If the patient has many lumps, are they the same? If the patient has had this before, what happened to it the last time, and what did the doctor say it was? Does it come periodically (for example, with every menstrual cycle)?
- *What do you think it is?* This is an important question, since the answer may be "Cancer, doctor". You are then aware of the patient's anxieties. You may be able to reassure the patient even if you do not know the exact diagnosis. For example, you may be able to reassure a 20-year-old girl with a painful breast lump that breast cancer is rare at her age and usually is not painful.

History of a Pain

Again, there are only a few questions you need to remember:
- Where is the pain?
- What is the nature of the pain?
- How did the pain start and what has happened to it since?
- What relieves and what exacerbates the pain?
- Are there any associated symptoms?
- Have you ever had this before?
- What do you think it is?

As seen with the questions for the history of a lump, this set of questions can apply to any pain, whether cardiac in origin or due to appendicitis. We now explore these questions in more detail.

- *Where is the pain?* Remember that visceral pain is referred along the somatic nerves; for example, diaphragmatic irritation is felt at the shoulder, and early appendicitis is felt around the umbilicus.
- *What is the nature of the pain?* This includes character, severity and radiation. Colicky pains feel like the contents of a tube are being squashed or pushed forward. They originate from a hollow viscus, and usually come and go in a regular pattern. Severity is difficult to standardise, since everyone has a different threshold of pain, but something like "The pain is worse than labour pains" or "This is the worst pain I have ever had" is often helpful.

- *How did the pain start and what has happened to it since?* This includes onset, progression and end. Was the onset sudden or gradual? Has the pain got better or worse since it started? Does it come and go? How is it now compared to when it started? It is sometimes helpful to get the patient to draw a graph of the pain against time.
- *What relieves and what exacerbates the pain?* Asking the patient for aggravating or relieving factors often draws a blank and you may have to ask more direct questions in this context. For example: "Does the pain want to make you writhe about or lie very still?" Classically, colicky pains make patients move about trying to get comfortable, whereas if there is inflammation involving the peritoneum then moving about makes the pain worse. This distinction is helpful in differentiating biliary colic, where the patient may be moving about during an episode, from cholecystitis, where the patient will tend to lie still.
- *Are there any associated symptoms?* Again, this will depend on the cause and site of the pain. For example, nausea, vomiting and signs of sympathetic stimulation all go with cardiac pain. Anorexia, weight loss, change in bowel habit and maybe rectal bleeding would be suggestive of bowel cancer.
- *Have you ever had this before?* If the patient has had this pain before they can usually tell you if this feels the same as the last episode. For example, an alcoholic with repeated episodes of acute pancreatitis, or an angina sufferer with a myocardial infarction. Ask about the patient's past medical history and what drugs the patient is taking.

Answering a Question

By the time finals come along, almost everyone knows how to answer a viva question with the same boring words: "I would take a thorough history, examine the patient and investigate according to my findings…" The examiner hears this statement time after time after time, and when the candidate cannot back it up with something more substantial, the examiner, rightly, might be disappointed.

A better approach which will make you stand out from the rest of the candidates is to control the examiner with your response. So, if for example you are asked how you would manage someone with a breast lump, you could say, "In taking the history I would find out about the history of the lump and ask in particular for risk factors for breast cancer or for factors suggestive of benign breast disease." The examiner might then ask, "And what are the risk factors for breast cancer?", or they might stay quiet in which case you would continue: "On examination I would inspect the breasts, followed by palpation, examining the normal side first, etc. My investigations would then be tailored to my findings from the history and examination, but should involve an imaging technique plus or minus a fine-needle aspiration. The patient would then require counselling about the disease, and treatment could be divided into medical and surgical options (which can be subdivided into curative and palliative)."

This is not meant to give you the full answer — it only highlights the approach you could use (the correct answer can be found in the chapter on breast surgery). What this answer shows is that you are thinking properly and not merely giving stereotypical responses. If the examiner wants to test you further they may then go on: "Good, so tell me what questions you would like to ask in taking the history of this lump." This way, you force the examiner into asking you questions that you want to hear, and hence you are always one step ahead. Likewise, if the examiner asks you for the complications of thyroidectomy, do not spend too much time on the general complications; rather, use a simple sentence like "Any operation has both general and specific complications and each can be divided into immediate, early and late. The specific complications of thyroidectomy are ..." If the examiner wishes to know the general complications they can then ask you for them. Answering in this way shows that you understand the question being asked.

It may be possible to give an adequate performance even when you are unsure of the exact diagnosis. A clear history or good clinical examination technique will go a long way towards persuading the examiners that you should pass. Often, if you have accurately reported the history and physical signs, the examiners will give you a hint towards the correct diagnosis if you do not get it immediately.

2

FLUID BALANCE AND PARENTERAL NUTRITION

Ian Nesbitt

During your first night on call as a doctor, it is almost certain that you will be asked to write up intravenous (IV) fluids. Fluid balance is one of the most important subjects in medicine. Sadly, it is a subject that is poorly covered in most textbooks and so in this chapter we start from first principles to help you understand and remember the topic.

BASIC FACTS

The human body is composed of approximately two-thirds water. The contribution of water to body weight depends on how much fat you carry, because fat contains very little water. People gain fat as they grow older. Women also tend to have a greater proportion of fat. Therefore women and the elderly will have a smaller proportion of total body water.

If we assume body water is 60% of our weight, then a 70 kg man will carry 42 l of water. Of this 42 l, two thirds (28 l) will be intracellular (ICF) and one third (14 l) will be extracellular (ECF). The extracellular fluid is subdivided into plasma (3 l), interstitial fluid (ISF, an aquatic habitat for the cells, about 10 l) and transcellular fluid (CSF, e.g. ocular, peritoneal and synovial fluids, about 1 l).

Osmotic pressure is the pressure needed for reverse osmosis (through a semi-permeable membrane, i.e. a cell wall). Simply put, it is the ability of a solute to attract water. Oncotic pressure, on the other hand, is the pressure exerted by proteins to draw fluids back in.

The osmolalities (reflecting the osmotic pressure) of the ICF and the ECF are similar although the main cation in the ECF is sodium, whereas in the ICF it is potassium. Fluid distribution between the ECF and the ICF is governed by changes in the osmotic pressure. This means that isotonic fluid (which has the same osmolality as plasma) administered into the plasma will not easily enter the ICF, since there is no difference in the osmolality.

Within the ECF, fluid distribution between the plasma and the ISF is governed by Starling forces (i.e. hydrostatic pressure which pushes fluid out of the blood vessels and oncotic pressure which sucks fluid back in). Therefore, fluid administered into the plasma will increase the hydrostatic pressure and dilute the oncotic pressure until the fluid is evenly distributed throughout the ECF (see Figure 2.1).

TYPES OF FLUID

Crystalloids are essentially electrolytes in water. Because they have no large molecules (and thus have no oncotic pressure) they are easily distributed to the extracellular spaces and so can be used as maintenance fluids. Examples of crystalloids are normal saline (which is isotonic = 0.9% saline) and 5%

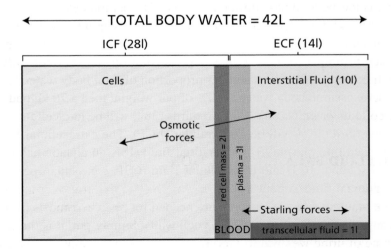

Figure 2.1.   Distribution of fluids within the body spaces.

dextrose (which is hypotonic). There is also a solution called Hartmann's solution, which contains lactate, potassium and calcium in addition to sodium chloride, and is therefore described as "physiological".

Colloids contain larger molecules which stay in the circulation for longer. They increase the intravascular oncotic pressure and thus can draw fluid back into the circulation. They are good for maintaining blood pressure, although, like crystalloids, they have no oxygen-carrying capacity. Examples of such colloids are Haemaccel® and Volplex®, both of which contain gelatine.

Why is this important? Well, if for example one gave 1 l of isotonic saline intravenously, it would initially only be distributed into the ECF (which includes the plasma). As plasma makes up only 3 l of the ECF which is 14 l, only 3/14 of the isotonic saline or 214 ml would remain in the plasma (the distribution takes minutes). In contrast, 1 l of 5% dextrose (which is hypotonic and so initially dilutes the ECF relative to the ICF) administered intravenously would be equally distributed throughout the body, and so 3/42 of 1 l or 70 ml would remain in the plasma. However, of 500 ml of a colloid given intravenously, all of it will stay in the plasma initially as there is no change in osmotic pressure and so there is no distribution into the cells (ICF). A transfusion of plasma or blood will also remain in the intravascular space, because the particle size (of proteins or cells) is too large to pass through the vascular membranes.

Although this idealised situation is not always entirely accurate when translated to the clinical environment, it allows a basic understanding of the key principles of fluid management, and demonstrates that different situations require different types of fluid replacement. For example, you can see why crystalloid preparations are of little use in acute blood loss, and colloids or blood are likely to be more appropriate.

THE FLUID BALANCE EQUATION

The simplest way to think about fluid balance is that it is an equilibrium where input must equal output. In order to live we must excrete all of our waste products. The main route for this is via the kidneys. The minimum volume of urine we need to produce in order to be healthy is about 1 l a day (0.5–1 ml/kg/h). This is the minimum obligatory volume of urine

(MOVU) to dissolve waste products. If less urine than this is produced, the patient is oliguric; and if no urine is produced, anuric.

At rest we also have other fluid losses that we are unaware of; these are called insensible water losses. Insensible losses occur from the lungs and in faeces, which amount to about 500 ml, and from the skin by sweating, which is also about 500 ml. If we add the MOVU to the insensible losses then our minimum daily fluid replacement is about 1.5–2 l.

This figure, however, relates to a healthy adult at rest; the requirements will go up with activity. In view of this we usually estimate that the average healthy adult will require about 3 l of fluids a day (Figure 2.2).

As well as water, we lose about 60 mM potassium and 100 mM sodium per day; these salts will also need replacing. In a normal person, large amounts of fluid are recycled in the body and must be accounted for in the so-called equilibrium. These include gastric juice

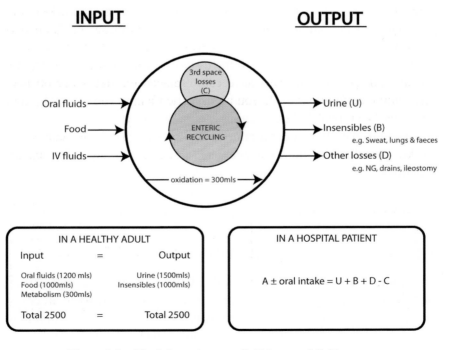

Figure 2.2.   The balance between fluid input and fluid output.

(3–4 l), bile (about 1 l) and intestinal secretions (3–4 l). This enteric recycling accounts for about 8 l/day and is mostly reabsorbed further down the GI tract.

It is common sense that any fluid and electrolyte losses must be replaced if we are to remain in equilibrium. This is usually achieved by our daily dietary intake of food and drink, although a small proportion of water is derived as a by-product of metabolism. When patients come into hospital they may be unable to have sufficient oral fluid intake either because they are nil by mouth (for example, perioperatively) or because they are unwell or vomiting.

Such patients require intravenous fluids and these can be any of the available crystalloid preparations. As highlighted above, the average adult will need about 3 l a day. This amount of dextrose saline would do (each 1 l bag contains 30 mM sodium). Another method would be to give 1 l of normal saline (containing 150 mM sodium) and 2 l of 5% dextrose. The dextrose is quickly metabolised, leaving water (note that giving 3 l of water intravenously would cause red cell haemolysis due to the osmotic gradient across the red blood cell membranes). In either of these two methods you have replaced 3 l of water with either 90 or 150 mM sodium. If you add 20 mM potassium to each 1 l bag (some bags come with this already added), then you will have also replaced the necessary 60 mM potassium (see Figure 2.3). If you request each bag to run over 8 h, then the 3 l will last the full day.

In cases where patients are on fluids for several days, it is inadvisable to prescribe dextrose saline alone, because after a few days of replacing

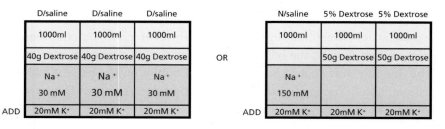

	D/saline	D/saline	D/saline			N/saline	5% Dextrose	5% Dextrose
	1000ml	1000ml	1000ml			1000ml	1000ml	1000ml
	40g Dextrose	40g Dextrose	40g Dextrose	OR			50g Dextrose	50g Dextrose
	Na⁺	Na⁺	Na⁺			Na⁺		
	30 mM	30 mM	30 mM			150 mM		
ADD	20mM K⁺	20mM K⁺	20mM K⁺		ADD	20mM K⁺	20mM K⁺	20mM K⁺

TOTAL = 3000mls + 90 mM NA⁺ + 60 mM K⁺   TOTAL = 3000mls + 150 mM NA⁺ + 60 mM K⁺

Figure 2.3.   Typical daily requirement of intravenous fluids; two alternative regimens.

too little sodium, the patient could well become hyponatraemic. This is easily avoided by adding normal saline to every third bag.

These are the standard regimens given to most normal adults. They are a reasonable starting point, but require modification depending on patient response to initial therapy. There are, of course, many exceptions to the rule, including the following.

The Postoperative Period

The metabolic response to the stresses of surgery involves a rise in various hormones, including circulating catecholamines, ADH, and stimulation of the hypothalamic-pituitary-adrenal axis, cortisol and aldosterone. The overall result of these is the renal conservation of salt and water, with somewhat increased losses of potassium and hydrogen ions. These effects usually last for about 24–48 h.

Despite the high potassium losses in the urine, the serum potassium is usually maintained or may even transiently rise, through release of cellular contents by damaged tissues. Therefore, unless serum potassium levels are very low, it is probably best to avoid potassium supplements on the first day or so postoperatively.

In addition, since water is being retained it is usual to reduce the fluid replacements to about 2 l on the first postoperative day, especially in patients prone to heart failure.

It is important to remember that a patient going to theatre is likely to have starved for several hours beforehand and may not have been given any fluids intraoperatively or whilst in recovery.

This patient will probably need extra fluids to maintain the fluid balance equilibrium. It is easy to see why one cannot rely on standard regimens when calculating how much fluid to give someone and so urine output may be the best indicator, aiming for greater than 50 ml/h. The nursing staff should document urine output on the patient's observation charts. Young, fit adults can usually tolerate excess fluids, so as long as the urine output is satisfactory, you are probably doing fine. The minimum urine output is about 30 ml/h (remember the MOVU). Obviously the urea and electrolytes can be checked, to help assess renal function.

Third-Space Losses

As mentioned before, about 8 l of secretions per day are reabsorbed in the bowel. A patient who has undergone abdominal surgery is likely to have a transient ileus postoperatively, where the bowel temporarily stops working. In such patients this is usually due to mechanical handling of the bowel, although any patient can suffer a transient ileus due to an electrolyte disturbance or even the effects of anaesthesia, especially if opiates are used. When an ileus is present, the fluid secreted into the bowel simply lies there and is not reabsorbed completely. These third-space losses mean that the patient effectively has a reduced volume of the ECF, and hence is fluid depleted. In such patients, extra fluid needs to be given to allow for the third-space losses. Unfortunately, you will not know how much extra fluid is needed and so must rely on urine output as an indicator. You will usually notice a sudden diuresis on day 2 or 3 postoperatively, explained by recovery from the ileus and reabsorption of the fluids from the bowel.

Similarly, in pancreatitis, patients can lose several litres of fluids rich in electrolytes and plasma proteins into the peritoneal cavity. Really, the only way to effectively gauge these losses is by vigorous replacement to maintain the urine output and to correct any electrolyte disturbances according to the daily U&E. If after two days 10 l have been put in with only 3 l of urine produced, then assuming 1–2 l of insensible losses, this equates to about 5–6 l of fluid sequestered into the peritoneal cavity.

Other Losses

If a patient has a nasogastric tube or a wound drain or is draining via a fistula, these losses need to be calculated daily and replaced (usually as normal saline) in addition to the standard losses.

Ileostomy patients can have huge losses, especially several days postoperatively. It is advisable to assess the ileostomy output at least twice daily, replacing these fluids and electrolytes accordingly to prevent acute dehydration.

Patients with pyrexia require more fluids. One can lose 3 l, maybe more, in certain circumstances. A rough estimate is to increase the fluid replacement by 10% for each degree of fever. Similarly, losses through vomiting or diarrhoea need replacing; remember that large-intestinal juices contain high concentrations of potassium and gastric juice contains lots of hydrogen ions.

Heart or Liver Failure

In heart or liver failure, because the renin-angiotensin system is already working overtime, conserving sodium, you should avoid giving fluids which contain sodium. Hence, you should mainly use 5% dextrose in these patients.

In heart failure, the patient is fluid overloaded, the usual cause in surgical patients being poor management of the fluid balance by the doctor. If you look at the fluid balance charts you will probably see a positive balance over the previous few days. Therefore, you will need to reduce the input, maybe even stop the fluids altogether and consider diuretics. Obviously, you should examine the patient regularly, measure their jugular venous pressure (JVP), listen to their chest and watch for oedema. Very sick patients on the ward may have a central venous pressure (CVP) line, and this makes the assessment of these patients a little easier. Ask the nursing staff to chart the patient's daily weight as this will help in monitoring progress.

Acute Renal Failure

This can be prerenal (e.g. hypovolaemia), renal (e.g. acute tubular necrosis) or postrenal (e.g. a blocked catheter). After surgery both pre- and postrenal causes are the commonest, and so should be looked for and treated first. If the patient is fluid depleted, this may be dealt with simply by correcting the dehydration. Look over the fluid balance charts from the previous days to decide whether the patient is in negative fluid balance. If you think that a renal cause is likely you should avoid potassium loads, stop any drugs that may affect renal function (such as NSAIDS, ACE inhibitors, etc.) and involve the renal team in the management early on. Without wishing to put words in their mouths, usually they advise replacing the previous days' output plus 500 ml to cover insensible losses. Alternatively one could measure the hourly urine output and replace 100% of this every hour.

In summary, input should equal output unless these exceptions apply. Look over the fluid balance charts (remember to bear in mind that in practice these could be inaccurate) and the daily weight charts. Assess the patient's state of hydration (dry lips, skin turgor, etc.) and check their blood results for renal function and haematocrit. Finally, do not forget the temperature, both of the patient and of the room.

We have deliberately gone into a lot of details on this subject, perhaps more than you need to know to pass your finals. This is because it is not really a topic that one can waffle about in the exam — either you understand the principles or you do not.

BLOOD TRANSFUSION

Blood transfusion is indicated for patients with anaemia, especially in the acute situation (e.g. active haemorrhage), although many chronic diseases also result in anaemia which may require transfusion. Unlike crystalloids and colloids, red cell transfusion increases the oxygen-carrying capacity of blood. The haemoglobin value which triggers transfusion will vary depending on the clinical context (increasingly, a trigger level of 7–9 g/dl is accepted as safe in many patient groups). A single unit of red cell concentrate (packed red cells) typically contains about 250–300 ml of concentrated blood (with a haematocrit of 0.6, rather than the normal 0.35) and will raise a patient's haemoglobin level by just under 1 g/dl.

Generally, transfusing one unit at a time and rechecking the Hb after each unit allows for an appropriate use of packed red cells.

Although blood is a drug, and transfusion has many potential hazards, the greatest risk is in misidentifying the patient, either through sample labelling errors when taking blood for cross-match or when actually connecting the bag of blood to the patient. Special care must therefore be taken at all times with blood transfusion.

Blood products (fresh frozen plasma, cryoprecipitate, platelets and other clotting factors) are used for particular indications. Fresh frozen plasma (FFP) was previously used for reversal of warfarin overdose, but specific drugs (prothrombin complex concentrate) now exist for this purpose, so FFP is used principally for the treatment of other combined coagulopathies. The dose used is typically four units at a time, guided by coagulation tests. Under some circumstances (e.g. major haemorrhage), large quantities of blood and FFP may be required, along with additional aids to clotting (platelets and cryoprecipitate).

The exact thresholds for the use of each product should be discussed with your seniors and haematologists (for example, a platelet count as low as $5 \times 10^9/l$ may be acceptable in some chronic medical conditions, but in acute surgical or trauma situations patients probably should have platelet counts above $50–100 \times 10^9/l$). Cryoprecipitate is typically given when plasma fibrinogen falls below 1 g/l.

NUTRITION

Patients who are malnourished are prone to many complications, such as delayed wound healing, muscle weakness and an increased tendency to infection. There is evidence that patients with poor nourishment prior to surgery will benefit from preoperative supplementation and do better after their operation. One caveat is that intervention must be for a reasonable period of time (more than ten days), in order to be of significant benefit.

There are lots of reasons why hospital patients become malnourished. They may have a decreased appetite due to the illness itself. They may have increased nutritional demands or their digestion may be impaired. Another reason could be due to the hospital stay itself, i.e. dislike of hospital food, being rushed off for an X-ray or ultrasound at noon, or being nil by mouth.

If oral intake is not anticipated within 7–10 days after surgery, then nutritional support is indicated (perhaps five days in a previously malnourished patient). The main indication for preoperative nutritional support is severe malnourishment (greater than 10% weight loss).

Nutritional support can vary from mere supplementation of vitamins, or protein in a high-protein diet, to a complete replacement of all essential foodstuffs. In this section, we only cover the latter.

Enteral vs. Parenteral Nutrition

Enteral diets are those given via the gut, including oral intake. Obviously the ideal situation is one where the patient takes in all the required nutrition orally; if this is not possible then enteral feeding is the next option. This involves passing the food into the gut, allowing it to be absorbed normally, either through a nasogastric tube or, if required for longer periods, via a gastrostomy or jejunostomy.

Parenteral nutrition bypasses the gut and involves a specialised feed directly into the patient's bloodstream. Parenteral nutrition may be used as a supplement to enteral feeding and it is usually given through a cannula in a peripheral vein. Alternatively, total parenteral nutrition (TPN) can be used to deliver the complete nutritional requirements. As TPN has a high osmolality it is toxic to veins and is usually given via a central line. The buzzwords to use would be "a small cannulae into a large vein with a high rate of blood flow". Hence a central venous line is usually used. For longer-term use, a Hickman line is preferred, which is a modified central line usually tunnelled under the skin to make it more secure and has a Dacron® cuff to prevent infection from entering. Unfortunately, parenteral feeding has some complications, including an increased risk of infection.

- It is common to be called to see a patient with parenteral feeding who has recently spiked a temperature. Obviously your management would be as for any pyrexia (see p. 38); however, if you suspect that the feed is the likely source of the infection, the correct thing to do is to stop the feed. If indeed this is the cause, then the temperature usually settles quickly, despite the fact that the central line is still *in situ* and may be infected. It appears that the running feed may be responsible for introducing the bugs from the infected line into the bloodstream. The central line will, however, probably need to be removed and replaced.
- Another complication of parenteral feeding is villous atrophy in the gut. Since the gut luminal cells (enterocytes) derive their nutrition from the lumen, long periods of rest can lead to atrophy. This makes the gut wall more permeable to bacterial flora and there is evidence that this can increase the risk of translocation of bacteria into the bloodstream.
- Electrolyte imbalances are likely and therefore the U&E should be checked daily and adjusted accordingly.

- Hyperglycaemia is another problem and the patient may need to be given insulin temporarily whilst on TPN. Other disturbances of liver function are common (possibly because of fatty infiltration of the liver) and a cholestatic picture may be seen with raised alkaline phosphatase, hence liver function tests (LFTs) should be performed every few days. Other electrolytes such as phosphate and magnesium should also be regularly checked.
- The take-home message must be that parenteral feeding should be reserved for patients in whom enteral feeding is impossible, such as patients with short gut syndrome, where large pieces of their gut have been surgically removed. Otherwise enteral feeding should be your first choice.

Requirements

- *Water.* See section on fluid balance; roughly 2–3 l per day.
- *Energy.* About 1800 calories per day. This is given as a mixture of carbohydrates and fats, roughly in a ratio of two thirds to one third respectively (but can be up to 50–50).
- *Nitrogen.* About 14 g per day in protein, but the requirement may change (8–20 g/day) according to the metabolic state.
- *Vitamins.* Fat-soluble vitamins are stored and so the levels should be carefully adjusted to avoid overdose. Water-soluble vitamins being excreted can be given more generously.
- *Minerals.* Sodium, potassium, calcium, magnesium, phosphate, etc.
- *Trace elements.* Zinc, copper, iron, selenium, iodide, etc.

The management of nutrition should be multidisciplinary, including the surgeon, the dietician, the pharmacist who makes up the feed, the nurses who actually administer it, and, if possible, the patient and their relatives. Parenteral feeds are usually made up into a single, complete, sterile 3 l bag (even if it contains only 2 l) in the pharmacy department according to the specific requirements of the individual patient.

The most important step is the connection of the feed to the patient as this is when infection is likely to occur, and hence it should be a sterile procedure.

Monitoring and assessment of nutritional status are best done on a clinical basis. The patient's appearance and weight are the best indicators. Other anthropometric measurements, such as skinfold thickness, are not ideal but may be of benefit in monitoring progress.

Daily measurement of albumin is pointless, since its half-life is long (about 21 days) and its level can be altered for many other reasons. However, it is helpful in long-term monitoring.

Transferrin is better than albumin in the short term, but probably the best day-to-day biochemical measurement is prealbumin (a liver protein), which is a good marker of nutritional status. Obviously, electrolytes should be measured daily and LFTs should be checked every few days.

Finally, of much amusement on ward rounds are the other markers of nutrition, such as grip strength and stool length — but as to who measures these, let alone how, I leave to your imagination.

3

PRE- AND POSTOPERATIVE MANAGEMENT

Ian Nesbitt and Andy Goldberg

Increasingly, preoperative assessment takes place in a preassessment clinic (PAC) a week or more before surgery. This provides a highly structured, comprehensive and efficient way to appropriately investigate and prepare patients for elective procedures. Even so, there will be many occasions when you are a surgical house officer (or F1) when patients bypass the PAC, e.g. emergency admissions. Part of your preoperative role will then be to clerk the patients and prepare them for the theatre or investigation.

A clerking consists of taking the history of the presenting complaint, past medical history, drug history (including allergies), family history and social history. You should then examine the patient fully, looking first at their general health and whether they are fit enough for the operation, and if not you should be thinking of ways to optimise their health, such as using preoperative nebulisers for an asthmatic. The clerking also allows other problems to be picked up.

If, when the patient arrives at the ward, you feel that the initial diagnosis has changed, you should inform a senior colleague before the operation is booked. For example, if a patient was admitted for an excisional biopsy of a lymph node that has completely disappeared when you examine the patient, you should inform your consultant as the operation might need to be cancelled.

In the main, appropriate investigations should be performed before surgery and this is often a good question for a viva examination. For example, before a laparoscopic cholecystectomy is performed, the patient should have had an ultrasound to confirm the presence of gallstones, as well as a set of liver function tests.

You should discuss the order of patients on the operating list with the operating surgeon. Usually children are placed first on the list, as this is nicer for the child and the parents; also they find it hard to go without food for long periods. Diabetics also should be put at the beginning of the list, in order to best manage their blood sugar levels.

If special equipment is needed in the theatre, such as an image intensifier for X-rays or laparoscopic equipment, then these should be discussed with the theatre staff (and radiographers) the day before.

Specialist nurses that have expertise in certain areas, such as breast disease, wound management and stomas, should be involved preoperatively in all appropriate cases. For example, a patient who is likely to need a colostomy or ileostomy should be seen by the stoma nurse specialist several days before the operation. This allows the specialist nurse to carry out patient education (i.e. to answer any questions and worries) and also to mark where the stoma will be sited (note that the patient should be standing, so as to position it in the most appropriate place). The surgical site should be marked with a permanent marker.

COMORBIDITY

Many patients have problems other than the one that is being operated upon. These may be social and may need a social work or occupational therapy referral. For example, if the patient has difficulty climbing stairs and there is no lift, then there may be a need to arrange for a stair lift or rehousing into ground floor accommodation.

The patients may have intercurrent medical problems such as diabetes, hypertension or chronic obstructive pulmonary disease (COPD). They may also be on drugs such as steroids or anticoagulants. When clerking the patient you should be looking out for these, and if you think they may affect the operation, then you should inform the anaesthetist or the consultant in charge of the patient.

Tests you should consider preoperatively include blood tests, such as a full blood count, a sickle cell screen if at risk (this includes anyone of Afro-Caribbean origin), and either a group and save or cross-match. You should cross-match any patient at risk of blood loss extensive enough to need replacing — many hospitals have agreed on policies for how much to cross-match for different operations, so you should ask your consultant for a copy of such a policy document. The blood is kept in the refrigerator ready for use. If it is not used it goes back to the blood bank for storage.

A young, healthy person, in general, requires no preoperative investigations, but if you are unsure you should ask the anaesthetist what they would like performed (e.g. some anaesthetists like to have a recent full blood count on all females of childbearing age). The National Institute for Health and Clinical Excellence (NICE) in the UK has issued guidelines on preoperative investigation and these are available on the Internet. If the patient is hypertensive or on diuretics then a urea, creatinine and electrolytes test to assess renal function must be performed. An electrocardiogram (ECG) is necessary on anyone who is hypertensive or has a history of heart disease. In many hospitals the requirement is to order an ECG and chest X-ray (CXR) as a baseline on the elderly (aged over 60), but check the policy in your hospital. The management of medical problems in surgical patients is essentially the same as that you read about in medical textbooks. We will, however, cover just a few important topics.

DIABETES

Diabetics have an increased incidence of perioperative complications. The stress of surgery can lead to an increased production of catabolic hormones, such as glucagon and catecholamines, which antagonise the action of insulin, making control more difficult, especially as the patient will also be nil by mouth. These patients are at an increased risk of infection (wound, chest, intravenous access sites and urine), peripheral vascular disease, pressure sores and ischaemic heart disease.

The aim is to maintain the patient's blood sugar level between 5 and 9 mmol/l. Preoperatively you should carry out a urine dipstick test to check for protein, send a blood sample to the laboratory for a blood glucose test, check the electrolytes and creatinine, and order an ECG. Most hospitals have a diabetic team available for advice, but the principles of management are outlined overleaf.

Management depends on the types of diabetes.

Insulin-Dependent Diabetics

For anything other than minor surgery it is probably best to put these patients on an insulin sliding scale to establish good control. This means they are on a drip of dextrose or dextrose saline (as they are not eating), together with a continuous infusion of fast-acting insulin (Actrapid). The rate of infusion of insulin will depend on their blood sugar level, which can be monitored by hourly BM stix (a finger-prick testing stick specific for glucose).

If the BM is low the infusion is decreased, and if the BM is high the insulin rate can be increased. It is important that you add potassium to each bag of fluids you give, since the insulin causes cellular uptake of potassium and can lead to hypokalaemia. Sliding scale regimens differ in different hospitals and you should try to get hold of the sliding scale protocol at your hospital. An example is given in Table 3.1.

An alternative to the sliding scale is to mix the dextrose, potassium and insulin in a single bag (generally 500 ml of 10% dextrose with 10 mmol KCl and 10 u Actrapid). This is infused at 80 ml/h, and the whole bag is changed with differing amounts of insulin depending on the BM values. This mixed bag is safer than a sliding scale, since the patient cannot receive an unopposed insulin infusion, but is more work for staff, as they have to change complete bags if BM control is poor rather than just altering the rate of insulin infusion.

Diabetics Controlled with Oral Hypoglycaemics

On the morning of the operation, omit the dose of oral hypoglycaemic. This can be resumed once the patient starts eating postoperatively. The BM should be measured, and if very high can be brought down by small doses of subcutaneous soluble insulin (e.g. six units of Actrapid). If this fails to control the sugar level or in the case of major surgery, simply

Table 3.1.   Sliding Scale for Insulin

BM (mmol/L)	0–4	4–8	8–12	12–16	>16
Rate of insulin (unit/h)	0.5	1.0	2.0	4.0	6.0

convert the treatment to a sliding scale approach. Diabetics should ideally be first on the list, as the starting time is predictable and this allows better management of sugar levels.

Diabetics Controlled by Diet Alone

This situation rarely needs any special measures. Remember that provided they have not been given any insulin or oral hypoglycaemics, these patients cannot become hypoglycaemic (unless they have an insulinoma); if anything their sugar level will be high. A BM stix will tell you where you stand if you are worried. If you find their control is poor then you should refer the patients back to their diabetologist.

STEROIDS

Patients on steroids are liable to impaired healing and postoperative infections. Also, long-term use of corticosteroids can lead to adrenal insufficiency, where the adrenals are unable to secrete the increased glucocorticoids necessary in response to the stresses of surgery. This can lead to an Addisonian crisis. Patients who have been on long-term oral steroids should therefore be treated with perioperative steroids. This usually means intravenous hydrocortisone before and after the operation until the patient can resume oral intake.

CHRONIC OBSTRUCTIVE PULMONARY DISEASE (COPD)

Surgery and anaesthesia predispose patients to basal lung collapse (atelectasis) and chest infection. This is especially true of operations to the abdomen, since the patient may be in pain and therefore does not cough up the secretions. Any pre-existing respiratory disease, such as COPD, increases the risk of chest complications, as do smoking, obesity and old age.

Preoperatively, patients with pre-existing chronic airways disease need a CXR and lung function tests. You should also do a baseline blood gas analysis if hypoxia or carbon dioxide retention is suspected. You can assess the degree of reversibility of the airway disease by measuring peak flows before and after bronchodilators. If there is a degree of reversibility then prescription of bronchodilators may help optimise lung function.

Physiotherapy is an important modality in these patients and preoperative breathing exercises can help prevent a chest infection. Postoperatively, physiotherapy should be initiated early to help remove airway secretions, especially in abdominal operations. Smokers should be encouraged to stop smoking at least four weeks prior to elective surgery.

DEEP VEIN THROMBOSIS (DVT)

All surgical patients are at risk of DVT. In some hospitals, prophylaxis with subcutaneous low-molecular-weight heparin (LMWH) injections and thromboembolic deterrent (TED) stockings are given to all surgical patients, whereas other hospitals only give these to patients at medium-to-high risk of DVT. NICE has published guidance for the appropriate management of thromboembolic prophylaxis. For example, any patient in a plaster cast is recommended to be on some form of DVT prophylaxis for the whole time they are in plaster. You should look up the NICE guidelines and check the policy at your hospital. Risk factors for DVT include previous thrombosis (DVT or pulmonary embolus), long periods of immobility, pelvic or hip operations, obesity, cancer and use of the oral contraceptive pill. (Note that progestogen-only pills (mini-Pill) have a much lower risk than other combined pills.)

Intermittent limb compression is where an inflatable device is wrapped around the legs and periodically blown up, from the distal to the proximal end, encouraging venous return. Also available is low-molecular-weight heparin, which is thought to work on the antiplatelet factor antithrombin III and therefore has little effect on the intrinsic clotting cascade. In normal prophylactic doses LMWH does not require monitoring; it is longer-acting and thus only needs to be given once daily. LMWH is as effective as unfractionated heparin. Newer drugs, such as direct thrombin inhibitors, are also now available.

In most cases, early mobilisation in combination with one or more of the above options is acceptable.

ANTIBIOTICS

Antibiotic cover is necessary for surgery if there is an increased risk of infection. This could be due to patient-related factors or those related to the type of operation.

Contaminated operations, such as those where the bowel contents can leak out, carry a high risk of infection, as do operations where a prosthetic implant is used (e.g. joint or heart valve replacement), and antibiotics should always be given in these cases. An example of a patient-related factor is mitral valve disease and the subsequent risk of developing endocarditis.

We usually give prophylactic antibiotics intravenously at the induction of anaesthesia, so that blood levels are high during the operation. If a tourniquet is being used, then the antibiotics must be given before the tourniquet is inflated.

You should have a rough idea of which organisms are likely to be responsible for infection and which antibiotics should therefore be used. Most hospitals will have local antibiotic policies tailored to their specific patient groups and infection demographics. Check the policy at your hospital on what antibiotics are given and whether a single dose or three doses are given.

Close liaison with the microbiologists is sensible. A common question concerns methicillin-resistant *Staphylococcus aureus* (MRSA), which is an increasing problem in many hospitals. It is especially worrying when it infects patients with prosthetic implants such as hip replacements or vascular bypasses.

Operations Involving the Bowel

Organisms

The organisms are mainly Gram-negative bacilli, i.e. coliforms, but also faecal anaerobes (*Bacteroides*) and *Staph. aureus* from the skin. In the gut there is also *Enterococcus faecalis* (also known as *Streptococcus faecalis*), but this causes infection less commonly. In bile, the majority of infections are with gut bacteria, such as *Escherichia coli*, and less commonly, *Pseudomonas*, which is more difficult to treat.

Prophylaxis

We tend to use a cephalosporin to cover the Gram-positive organisms together with metronidazole to cover anaerobes. If you are concerned about *Strep. faecalis* you should add amoxycillin, as the cephalosporins do not cover this well. For operations on the biliary tree, such as a laparoscopic cholecystectomy, you could either use the same regimen as above or just use a cephalosporin alone, as most infections are with Gram-negative bacilli (mainly *E. coli*). One dose at induction is sufficient. For improved biliary penetration such as before and after an endoscopic retrograde cholangiopancreatogram (ERCP) or for ascending cholangitis, a broad-spectrum β-lactam such as piperacillin is often used. This also covers *Pseudomonas*.

Operations Involving Prosthetic Implants

Organisms

Skin organisms are usually responsible for infections. *Staph. aureus* is the commonest pathogen, but *Staph. epidermidis* and less commonly coliforms are also responsible.

Prophylaxis

Either a broad-spectrum cephalosporin or flucloxacillin can be used. Orthopaedic operations involving metalwork require a dose of intravenous antibiotics (usually a cephalosporin) at induction. In some hospitals this is all the microbiologists recommend. In others two further doses are also given. Check your hospital's antibiotic policy for local guidelines. The *British National Formulary* (BNF) is also a good place to obtain up-to-date information. Similarly, patients who have undergone valve replacements are usually given amoxycillin (or a cephalosporin) and gentamycin. If MRSA is a particular worry, then vancomycin may be used.

If ischaemic or necrotic tissue is involved then spores of *Clostridium tetani* may cause gas gangrene. Benzylpenicillin, to which the organism is highly susceptible, is the prophylaxis (and treatment) of choice against this (including penetrating wounds and open fractures).

The mnemonic "ABCD LMNOPs" is helpful for remembering all the possible options in preoperative management:

- A: Antibiotics/Anaesthetist
- B: Blood tests (including cross-match)/Bowel preparation
- C: Consent/CXR
- D: Drug chart/DVT prophylaxis
- E: ECG
- F: Fluids (especially if the patient is nil by mouth or vomiting)
- L: List (put in the operating list)/Lung function tests
- M: Mark the area or limb (this should be done by the operating surgeon)
- N: Notes should be written — documentation is vital
- O: Operating theatre staff (e.g. book special equipment/radiology)
- P: Physiotherapy (for the patient preoperatively as well as post-operatively)
- S: Specialist nurses (e.g. breast care or stoma care nurses)

POSTOPERATIVE MANAGEMENT

The role of the junior doctor in the postoperative period is to check that the patient has recovered from the anaesthetic, look at the observation charts and check the fluid balance. The operation note should have a section on specific postoperative management written by the surgeon, and is a guide that should be followed. For example, following a vascular graft operation, say, to the leg, you should always check the pulses, capillary refill and toe movement in the involved leg to ensure that the graft has not blocked off. Likewise, the anaesthetic chart usually has instructions for specific post-operative investigations, fluid management and analgesia, including epidural or intravenous patient-controlled analgesia (PCA) devices.

A common question in exams concerns complications of surgery.

Complications

All operations carry a risk of complications. These can be divided into general and specific complications. General complications include those pertaining to the anaesthesia itself and those that can occur after any operation, such as a chest infection or DVT. Specific complications are those that occur because of the individual operation itself, such as cutting a nerve.

You can subdivide this classification by time, into immediate complications, which occur within the first 24 hours; early, within the first week or so; late postoperative, occurring within the first month or so; and long-term.

General immediate complications include those due to the anaesthetic, such as direct trauma to the mouth and teeth when intubating, and rare reactions to the anaesthetic (inherited disorders or idiosyncratic reactions). Early complications include chest infections, urinary retention or infections, DVT and bed sores.

Specific complications depend on the nature of the operation and are dealt with in various chapters of this book. Two important specific complications are haemorrhage and wound infection and these will be discussed more here.

Haemorrhage

This can be divided into primary, reactionary and secondary haemorrhage.

Primary haemorrhage occurs during the operation, when a vessel is cut. Reactionary haemorrhage is when at the end of the operation the wound looks dry, but bleeding begins afterwards, when the patient's blood pressure and cardiac output rise to normal levels, presumably from vessels that were not properly ligated during the operation. Secondary haemorrhage, occurring several days after the operation, is usually attributed to infection that erodes through a vessel.

Wound Infections

These are most commonly caused by *Staph. aureus*, although coliforms such as *E. coli* are also important. Wound infection is more likely if

- The operation is dirty (e.g. abdominal surgery)
- The duration of the operation is long (greater than 2 h)
- The patient is more susceptible (e.g. old age, immunosuppression, diabetes)

Minor wound infections, with a little redness and slight discharge, are relatively common and usually need just simple measures, such as regular wound dressing and perhaps antibiotics. More severe infections, common after abdominal operations, usually occur in the first week or so. The wound looks inflamed and there may be cellulitis, discharge or localised abscess formation. The wound should be swabbed and maybe antibiotics started, but the correct treatment for an abscess is drainage. This may mean simply removing a few of the surgical clips and probing the wound, allowing the pus to discharge, or a further surgical procedure to open up the wound. The wound is then left to heal by secondary intention (i.e. to heal itself from within, with no further suturing).

Wound Dehiscence

This is an uncommon problem. It is usually due to an inadequate repair of the tissues (but infection, poor blood supply, malnutrition and steroids may all play a part in poor wound healing). Dehiscence usually occurs about a week after the operation. A warning sign is a serosanguinous discharge from the wound a few days before. The wound suddenly bursts open and in the case of a laparotomy the bowel protrudes outwards and is extremely alarming for the patient and nursing staff. Sterile, soaked swabs should be placed over the wound and the patient taken back to the theatre for repair.

Examples of general and specific complications pertaining to a gastrectomy are outlined in Table 3.2.

Table 3.2. General and Specific Complications Pertaining to a Gastrectomy

	Specific	General
Immediate	Haemorrhage	Broken tooth
(within 24 h)	Damage to nearby structures (e.g. spleen)	Anaphylaxis to anaesthetic drugs
Early	Paralytic ileus	Chest infection
(1st week or so)	Anastomotic leak	Urinary tract infection
	Infection	Pulmonary embolus
	Wound	DVT Bed sores
	Deep collection	
Late	Inability to eat normal-sized meals	Weight loss
(1st month or so)	Dumping syndrome	(combination of all of the complications)
	Steatorrhoea/diarrhoea	
Long-term	Recurrence of ulcer	Osteoporosis Anaemia
	Malignancy	Pernicious
		Iron-deficient

For further elaboration see Chapter 6. The general complications are pretty much the same for all operations. Try to draw up a list of the specific complications for other common procedures, such as a hip replacement or operations on the colon, thyroid and breast.

The commonest reasons that a junior doctor gets called to the ward are to write up fluids or to see a patient with postoperative pyrexia or poor urine output, so let's discuss these a little here.

POSTOPERATIVE PYREXIA

A small rise in temperature is common postoperatively. If the temperature spikes above 38 °C or persists, then you should consider and look for the seven Cs as potential causes. This is a common viva question.

• *Chest*	Chest infection
• *Catheter*	Urinary tract infection
• *Central venous pressure line*	Infected
• *Cannula*	Superficial thrombophlebitis (solved by removing the cannula)
• *Cut*	Wound infection
• *Collection*	Subphrenic or pelvic abscess (may indicate a failure of anastomosis)
• *Calves*	DVT (rumbling pyrexia in second postoperative week)

A chest infection is common postoperatively, especially in patients who smoke or have pre-existing poor respiratory function. Mucous secretions are not cleared; these then clog up the smaller bronchi, leading to collapse of the air spaces distal to the blockage (atelectasis). Inhaled organisms then infect the collapsed segments. In addition, thoracic and upper abdominal incisions cause pain and stop patients from coughing up the secretions, and so they are much more likely to have basal atelectasis and develop chest infections. These patients should therefore be given adequate analgesia, have vigorous physiotherapy and be encouraged to cough up the phlegm (ideally whilst holding their wounds — applicable for chest and abdominal wounds).

A deep collection, such as a subphrenic or pelvic abscess, can occur after the patient has had generalised peritonitis. The patient usually presents with general malaise, nausea, pain (a subphrenic abscess may also cause pain felt in the shoulder tip), swinging pyrexia and localised peritonitis.

A pelvic abscess often occurs 4–10 days postoperation, whereas a subphrenic abscess usually occurs a bit later, 7–21 days postoperation. Clinically, the patient appears to be recovering well, but then develops a fever and feels unwell. The white cell count may be raised and a collection is identified on ultrasound or CT. Treatment is by drainage, either percutaneously under ultrasound or CT guidance, or by an open procedure. A drain is usually left *in situ*.

A small anastomotic leak usually causes a localised abscess which becomes sealed off by the omentum and the bowel. Clinically the patient is slow to recover, but usually improves with intravenous antibiotics and fluids and delayed return to food. A larger anastomotic breakdown causes the patient to be very unwell, with anything from local peritonitis through to a rigid abdomen and septicaemia. The abscess needs to be drained, the peritoneal cavity washed out and the two ends of the failed anastomosis can be brought out as temporary stomas.

A diagnosis of DVT or pulmonary embolus (PE) in the first instance is usually a clinical one. A patient with DVT presents with pain and swelling of the calf. After a knee replacement diagnosis can be difficult as the leg is generally swollen anyway, but if the swelling has suddenly increased a couple of weeks after the operation then it is sensible to arrange a duplex ultrasound (or a venogram) to rule out DVT.

Pulmonary embolus usually presents with pleuritic chest pain (stabbing pain and worse on inspiration). The textbooks tend to describe the findings you would see in a massive PE, although more common are the smaller PEs where the findings are less impressive. Usually, the patient is tachycardic, maybe with a low-grade fever and tachypnoea, but may even be asymptomatic. The ECG usually shows sinus tachycardia (the classic S1Q3T3, which students know all about, occurs when there is a large amount of right heart strain, in a large PE, and is very rarely seen). The CXR may show a small area of linear atelectasis, but is helpful mainly in excluding other differential diagnoses. Blood gas analysis is essential and you would expect to find a low PO_2 (due to ventilation/perfusion mismatch) and perhaps a low PCO_2 due to hyperventilation. Examination of the calves may or may not reveal evidence of DVT. If DVT or PE is suspected, a heparin infusion or therapeutic doses of LMWH can be started before investigation but always check with a senior colleague before making any decisions, especially if the patient has had recent surgery.

To diagnose a PE you can request a ventilation/perfusion scan, although the gold standard is now CT pulmonary angiography.

Other less common causes for a fever include infective diarrhoeas, drug reactions and blood transfusion reactions.

If faced with a pyrexial patient you would obviously explore the history and examine the patient properly. In a viva situation you could answer along these lines: "I would listen to the chest, examine the abdomen, check the cannula sites, inspect the wound, etc... My investigations would depend on my clinical findings but may involve sending a urine specimen, a full blood count and blood cultures, sending wound swabs or the tip of the central line for culture etc."

DRAINS

Collections within a wound (especially if they contain blood) are the perfect medium for colonisation of bacteria and hence infection.

A drain can be used to remove anticipated collections within a wound, but should never be used as a substitute for adequate haemostasis at the time of surgery.

Drains can be closed or open. Closed drainage includes suction drainage (e.g. Redivac) where the collection is attracted into a container either by gravity or suction. This can then potentially reduce the risk of infection when used for large spaces or cavities, such as after a mastectomy or joint replacement. Drains are usually removed as soon as possible (usually 24–48 h) or as soon as the losses begin to tail off. Drains can also introduce infections and so they should not be left in place for longer than needed.

Open drainage (e.g. a piece of corrugated tubing with one end in the wound and the other in the dressing) allows small losses to escape from the wound. This is often employed in established abscesses after incision and drainage to allow any remaining collection a passage out of the wound. Some surgeons like to withdraw this type of drain in stages to allow the track to collapse behind it.

Other drains commonly asked about in exams include chest drains, T-tubes and percutaneous nephrostomies (discussed in the relevant sections).

POSTOPERATIVE POOR URINE OUTPUT

This is a common exam question, so it is best to develop a system to discuss it logically. Poor urine output can be classified as prerenal, renal or postrenal. The commonest causes of failure to pass urine postoperatively are postrenal.

Postrenal problems (commoner in males) include obstruction caused by a large prostate or a blocked catheter. Also the patient may find initiation of micturition difficult for the following reasons:

- Anticholinergic drugs or those with α-adrenergic effects (e.g. some anaesthetic drugs)
- Pain (e.g. after a hernia repair)
- Inhibition (e.g. because of strange surroundings or a nurse continually asking them if they have passed urine)
- Opiates or epidural anaesthetics

Once the bladder reaches a certain volume of distension it fails to function properly and the patient goes into retention. Benign prostatic hypertrophy is an important predisposition and these patients are more likely to go into retention.

Prerenal causes are due to renal hypoperfusion because of either hypovolaemia or heart failure and will not be covered here.

As for renal causes, acute postoperative renal failure is usually due to acute tubular necrosis and can be looked up in a medical textbook.

Junior doctors are commonly called to see patients who have failed to pass urine postoperatively. Often this will be a patient you have not met before. It is therefore worth spending a little time obtaining a history and reading the patient's notes. You should find out the type and date of

4

TRAUMA, SHOCK, HEAD INJURIES AND BURNS

Peter Smitham and Andy Goldberg

TRAUMA

Imagine yourself being faced with a multiply injured patient with trauma to the head, chest, abdomen and limbs. Where would you start? What if there were several injured patients — which would take priority?

The Advanced Trauma and Life Support (ATLS®)* course was developed following a tragedy. In 1976, an orthopaedic surgeon who was piloting his own plane over rural Nebraska crashed in a cornfield. His wife died instantly and three of his four children sustained critical injuries. When they were taken to the nearest medical facility, the surgeon was appalled at the poor quality of care that he and his family received and felt that a system was needed to improve the care of trauma patients.

Causes of Death in Trauma

There is a trimodal distribution of death following injury. The first peak occurs at the time of the injury, usually due to severe lacerations of the brain, heart or large blood vessels, and the patient is usually dead before

* Used/modified with permission from the American College of Surgeons Committee on Trauma (2008), *Advanced Trauma Life Support® Manual 2008*, 8th Edition (Chicago: American College of Surgeons).

arrival in casualty. Prevention by methods such as using seat belts, wearing crash helmets and following speed limits is the only effective way of reducing these deaths.

The second peak occurs within minutes to hours of the injury. Injuries such as a tension pneumothorax, blood loss and intracranial bleeds account for this peak. These deaths are potentially avoidable with immediate medical management.

The third peak of death occurs several days to weeks after the incident, due to sepsis and multiorgan failure. The care provided during the initial resuscitation and subsequent period directly affects the outcome of this group.

The concept behind ATLS® is to treat life-threatening injuries first and all other injuries in order of priority. Since a blocked airway kills within seconds this clearly should have first priority; likewise a tension pneumothorax will kill before bleeding from a wound.

The ATLS® approach is divided into a primary and a secondary survey. In the primary survey, life-threatening injuries are identified. In this chapter we look at assessment and resuscitation separately, although in reality they take place simultaneously (i.e. life-threatening injuries are treated as soon as they are identified). The secondary survey is a more thorough head-to-toe examination.

The patient is continuously re-evaluated until they are stable and a definitive care pathway can be instituted.

Primary Survey

As the patient arrives there is usually some history available — if not from the patient, then from witnesses or the ambulance crew. The vital signs from when first seen by the paramedics until the time of arrival in the A&E department should be noted.

The primary survey is a rapid evaluation; the mnemonic "ABCDE" can be used to allow one to think in an ordered and prioritised manner.

- A: Airway with cervical spine control
- B: Breathing and ventilation
- C: Circulation with haemorrhage control

- D: Disability
- E: Exposure and environment

A — *Airway with Cervical Spine Control*

In anyone with an altered level of consciousness or injuries above the clavicles, suspect a cervical spine injury. The patient's head should be supported by a hand on either side to prevent any movement (in-line manual immobilisation), and when possible a semi-rigid collar should be applied with two sandbags on either side of the head with tape across them to hold them in place.

The airway should be checked to see if it is patent or if there are signs of airway obstruction. Listen for noisy breathing, look for obvious facial trauma and inspect for foreign bodies.

B — *Breathing and Ventilation*

Assess the respiratory function. Inspect and palpate for tracheal deviation, expansion of the lungs and for any lacerations, rib fractures or flail segments. A flail chest, commonly asked about in exams, is a segment of the chest wall that, owing to multiple fractures, has no bony continuity with the rest of the thoracic cage. The flail segment moves paradoxically to the rest of the chest (i.e. it moves in on inspiration and out on expiration). The hypoxia that results is usually not due to the flail segment alone but more to the underlying contusion to the lung and hence mismatches between ventilation and perfusion.

C — *Circulation with Haemorrhage Control*

Assess the level of consciousness, pulse, blood pressure, respiratory rate, skin colour and capillary refill time (see p. 57). Hypotension following injury must be assumed to be due to hypovolaemia until proved otherwise.

During the primary survey any external severe bleeding points should be controlled by applying a sterile pressure dressing or a pneumatic splint. Tourniquets are usually avoided, as they cause crush injuries and distal ischaemia.

Internal bleeding should be suspected and you should examine systematically for all of the common causes, such as an intrathoracic or intra-abdominal bleed or a fractured pelvis and/or femur. A bleed into the cranial cavity will not by itself cause hypovolaemia.

D — *Disability*

This is a rapid neurological evaluation assessing the patient's level of consciousness and the pupil size and response to light. The mnemonic "AVPU" is used as a quick assessment of the patient's level of consciousness. If, for example, the patient responds only to pain, then the AVPU score is P.

- A: Alert
- V: responds to Verbal stimuli
- P: responds to Painful stimuli
- U: Unresponsive

The Glasgow Coma Scale (GCS) is a more detailed neurological evaluation that can be done during the primary survey although it takes a little longer, and because the life-threatening A, B and C take precedence in the primary survey the GCS may be performed in the secondary survey (see section on head injury for details).

A decreased level of consciousness may be due to many factors, including cerebral injury, hypoxia and shock. It may also be secondary to alcohol and drugs, although head injury, hypoxia and shock must be excluded first.

E — *Exposure*

Completely undress the patient (cut off the clothes as appropriate), inspect the entire skin surface for evidence of injury, such as bruising, abrasions or lacerations. A log roll should be performed with in-line cervical spine immobilisation (i.e. the head is supported and turned in line with the patient to prevent any displacement of the cervical spine). The entire vertebral column is palpated down to the coccyx for tenderness and a rectal examination is performed.

Imaging is an important part of the ATLS® system, and traditionally a trauma series would be taken on the cusp between primary and secondary surveys. The trauma series of X-rays included a lateral C-Spine, chest and pelvic X-ray. More recently, rapid spiral CT scans have significantly changed management and are preferred over plain radiographs in major trauma centres. The trauma series remains an important element of ATLS® management where rapid CT facilities are not available. An electrocardiogram (ECG) is also usually taken.

A nasogastric tube should be considered. (Note: This is contraindicated if a cribriform plate fracture is suspected as the tube could enter the cranial vault, and an orogastric tube may be used instead.) A urinary catheter should also be considered. (Note: During the rectal examination, a high-riding prostate or any sharp, bony, pelvic fragments might indicate a urethral transection which would mean transurethral catheterisation is contraindicated. Other signs suggesting a urethral injury: blood at the urethral meatus or a scrotal haematoma. If a urethral transection is suspected then a retrograde urethrogram can be performed and a suprapubic catheter might be needed.)

Once a full exposure has been performed it is important that the patient is covered to prevent hypothermia. This can develop rapidly due to shock, exposure and fluid resuscitation.

RESUSCITATION

As mentioned before, this is carried out simultaneously during the primary survey.

Airway

Every injured patient should receive supplemental oxygen; however, the airway must be patent and protected in all patients. There are five things you can do to ensure a patent airway; always start with simple measures, such as the chin lift, and progress through the following list until oxygenation is adequate. Apply an oxygen mask with a reservoir (to allow about 85% oxygen).

- *Chin lift or jaw thrust.* In the supine position the tongue naturally falls back, obstructing the hypopharynx. These procedures bring the tongue forward, opening up the airway. In the chin lift the chin is grasped between the first finger and the thumb. The chin is then lifted gently and brought anteriorly (being careful not to hyperextend the neck). In the jaw thrust manoeuvre the angles of the mandible are grasped by a hand on each side and the lower jaw is brought forward.

- *Guedel airway*. If breathing is still noisy, you can maintain the airway by inserting an oropharyngeal airway, such as a Guedel airway (an S-shaped plastic tube). The size should correspond to the distance from the centre of the patient's mouth to the angle of the jaw. It is sometimes put in upside down and rotated when it is past the tongue.
- *Nasopharyngeal tube*. If the patient is conscious and has a gag reflex, they will be unlikely to tolerate an oropharyngeal airway. In this case a nasopharyngeal airway can be tried, as it is better tolerated and less likely to induce vomiting. However, many conscious patients will not tolerate either and may need to be anaesthetised and intubated.
- *Intubation*. This is called a definitive airway, which means a tube is inserted into the trachea with a cuff inflated to prevent aspiration; the whole thing is secured with tape and oxygen is connected. A definitive airway can be an orotracheal tube, a nasotracheal tube or a surgical airway (see next item in the list). A definitive airway is needed if the patient is not breathing, if the patient is unable to maintain an airway with the previous measures, if there is impending airway compromise (as in inhalation injuries) or in a head injury requiring hyperventilation. It is important to be able to predict if the patient's airway is likely to be difficult to intubate. The ATLS® system has a method to help assess the patient's airway but you really don't need to know about it in detail for the purpose of your finals. More importantly, you should not attempt an intubation if it is beyond your skills. It is better to establish a patent airway with the use of simple methods rather than to rush ahead and attempt an intubation that may cause further damage if you are not confident. Since CO_2 is produced in the lungs you can confirm the tube is in the trachea by measuring the end-tidal CO_2 tension. If the tube was mistakenly placed into the oesophagus then the CO_2 gas pattern would be absent. Proper placement of the tube is also checked by listening for bilateral air entry (for example, if the tube is in the right main bronchus then no air entry will be heard on the left).

- *Surgical airway.* If you are unable to intubate (for example, in severe facial trauma) then a surgical airway is indicated. A tracheostomy is difficult to perform and is time-consuming, so a needle cricothyroidotomy can be performed instead by inserting a large-calibre cannula through the cricothyroid membrane into the trachea (feel for the Adam's apple, and move your finger downwards till you come to the first gap between the thyroid and cricoid cartilages). Oxygen is then connected to the airway.

A needle cricothyroidotomy will only buy a short amount of time and must be converted to a surgical cricothyroidotomy by widening the incision and placing a cuffed endotracheal tube into the space between the thyroid and cricoid cartilages. (If you are ever asked about the difference between a tracheostomy and a surgical airway, then note that a tracheostomy is placed into the trachea at about the level of the second or third tracheal ring and is a much longer procedure as the thyroid gland has to be divided and is therefore performed in theatre when the patient is stable.)

Breathing

The mnemonic "ATOMIC" has been used to list life-threatening chest injuries, which should be identified in the primary survey:

- A: Airway obstruction
- T: Tension pneumothorax
- O: Open pneumothorax
- M: Massive haemothorax (greater than 1500 ml)
- I: Intercostal disruption (some people modify the mnemonic to "ATOM FC", where F stands for "flail chest")
- C: Cardiac tamponade

A tension pneumothorax occurs when air enters the pleural space either from outside or from inside the lung. A one-way valve is formed by the pleura, which allows air to enter the pleural space during inspiration, but does not allow it to escape during expiration. The lung collapses, and the mediastinum and the trachea are deviated away from the affected side. The patient becomes very short of breath and cyanotic. The venous return to the heart is impaired and the signs are similar to those of cardiac tamponade, i.e. raised jugular venous pressure (JVP) and falling blood pressure (BP), but they can be differentiated by listening for breath sounds. The diagnosis is made clinically — a distressed, tachycardic patient has a deviated trachea, hyperresonance to percussion and absent breath sounds on the affected side. You should never see a chest X-ray on patients with a tension pneumothorax, as they should have been treated immediately before waiting for an X-ray to be taken. Treatment is by placing a cannula (Venflon) into the second intercostal space, midclavicular line, and hearing a hiss as the air escapes. Once this is performed the tension pneumothorax will be converted to a simple pneumothorax and the immediate threat to life is over. A chest drain should be inserted as soon as possible.

In an open pneumothorax, if the opening is approximately two thirds of the diameter of the trachea, then air passes through the wound in preference to the airway during inspiration (taking the route of least resistance). This is also called a sucking chest wound. The management is to close the wound with a sterile dressing taped on three sides to form a flap valve.

Insertion of a Chest Drain

A chest drain is inserted under aseptic technique anterior to the midaxillary line, in the fifth intercostal space. If possible (provided no cervical spine injury is suspected) have the patient sit up at 45° and place their hand behind their neck on the affected side to expose the field and open up the intercostal space.

If sitting up is not possible then the procedure should be performed with the patient supine. Again the arm on the affected side is placed behind the patient's neck. The area is prepared with antiseptic (e.g. Betadine) and draped. Some anaesthetic is infiltrated into the skin, subcutaneous tissues and down to the pleura. A 2 cm transverse incision is made in the fifth intercostal space (aiming above the rib as the intercostal bundle sits in the groove just below the rib). Blunt dissection is then performed down to the pleura with a pair of forceps which are pushed through the pleura into the pleural space.

A finger is placed in the hole and swept around to free any adhesions and create a space for the tube. A chest tube is inserted using a pair of forceps, usually French gauge 24–28 (if a haemopneumothorax exists a larger tube size, Fr 38, is usually used). The drain is fixed with a stitch and a purse-string or mattress suture is placed in the wound (to allow it to be closed when the drain is removed). The chest drain is connected to an underwater seal (this allows air to escape during expiration, but no air to enter on inspiration). Ensure that the underwater seal is below the patient, otherwise the water will enter the chest. Re-X-ray the patient after the procedure to ensure correct positioning of the tube.

If you are ever asked how you can check if a chest drain is blocked, a top tip is to ask the patient to cough and you will see bubbles escaping if it is patent.

Circulation (see p. 59)

Two large-bore cannulae should be inserted, one into each antecubital fossa, for all patients exposed to major trauma. Blood should be taken for a cross-match, a full blood count, and urea and electrolytes (U&E).

The ATLS® system recommends giving 2 l of warmed physiological fluids (Hartmann's or Ringer's lactate) immediately, although some surgeons in the UK often start colloids (such as Haemaccel) if there is definite blood loss, and indeed new research exploring permissive hypotension and early administration of tranexamic acid and clotting factors might pave the way for changes in practice the world over. Obviously it is important to get the blood as soon as possible. O negative blood (the universal donor) is used if necessary whilst awaiting the cross-match.

The most important thing is to recognise the signs of shock, and look for a cause. The chest, abdomen and pelvis are the likely causes if there is no obvious haemorrhage from a wound. A bleed into the abdomen causes distension and signs on examination such as tenderness, guarding and maybe absent bowel sounds. If intraperitoneal bleeding is suspected (say, in a stab wound) and the patient is shocked despite immediate resuscitation, then no time should be wasted and the patient should be taken straight to theatre for a laparotomy to "turn off the tap". If the findings on examination are equivocal and the patient is not unstable, then a diagnostic peritoneal lavage (DPL), ultrasound (FAST scan — Focused Assessment with Sonography for Trauma) or computed tomography (CT) scan can be performed. In FAST, a repeat ultrasound is required ideally after an interval of 30 minutes or so to exclude any progressive haemoperitoneum in patients with a slow bleeding rate. Although FAST scans have the advantage of being non-invasive and are rapid to perform they do have the disadvantage of being operator-dependent and may miss diaphragmatic or solid organ injuries.

An unstable fractured pelvis can cause profuse blood loss and Stage IV shock. The cause is usually venous bleeding. During the primary survey the chest and abdomen will have been examined for other causes of the shock. An orthopaedic surgeon can place an external fixator onto the pelvis, which usually stops the rapid blood loss (by tamponade; it also stops any shearing forces on the vessels).

Diagnostic Peritoneal Lavage (DPL)

For finals you probably just need to know that this involves an incision in the midline, below the umbilicus, and dissection down to the peritoneum, into which a catheter is placed.

A litre of normal saline is run into the peritoneal cavity. The bag is then placed on the floor and allowed to fill. If there is no obvious blood, then a sample of fluid is sent for microscopy to count the red blood cells. A urinary catheter and nasogastric tube must be inserted prior to the DPL in order to avoid damage to the stomach and bladder during the procedure. The findings of this procedure, however, are often equivocal.

Disability

See section on head injury (p. 62).

Exposure/Environment

The patient is completely exposed so that a full examination can be performed. In order to protect them from heat loss, both the patient and the resuscitation room should be heated. Methods for heating the patient include the use of warmed fluids and blood, and the use of blankets. A log roll may be performed here, or it may be performed in the secondary survey.

In the log roll procedure one person holds and turns the head and neck and three people roll the body. This allows the patient to be turned with in-line cervical spine immobilisation to examine the back of the body for any signs of trauma (stab wounds, bruising, abrasions), palpating for any tenderness. A rectal examination is also performed.

Secondary Survey

A quick history should be ascertained, from witnesses, family or the Paramedics. The mnemonic "AMPLE" is used for the following vital questions:

- A: Allergies
- M: Medication
- P: Past medical history
- L: Last ate or drank
- E: Events prior to the accident

The secondary survey is the head-to-toe or full examination. Check the head (eyes, ears, scalp — run your fingers through the hair), cervical spine, chest, abdomen, limbs, and perform a full neurological examination. If the log roll has not been performed in the primary survey, it should be performed here.

At the end of the secondary survey the patient should be re-evaluated by starting again at the ABCs. Once you are sure they are fully stabilised you can begin to make arrangements for definitive care (this usually means an admission).

Cervical Spine: X-Rays and Management

A cervical spine injury is almost always accompanied by pain in the neck; however, it is important to know that the absence of a neurological deficit does not rule out a fracture of the cervical spine. Under A for "airway" with cervical spine control, the neck should be immobilised. If a motorcycle helmet needs to be removed or intubation is required, these should be performed with in-line manual immobilisation. The ATLS® currently recommends a lateral shoot-through X-ray; however, current trends are moving towards CT scans in the emergency department within 15–30 minutes of admission, and the CT is used to exclude a C-Spine fracture.

Assessment of the Cervical Spine X-Ray

A common question in exams is how to assess a C-Spine X-ray. Although, as stated above, C-Spine X-rays may not be captured so often in major trauma centres nowdays, it is still important for you to know how to review this imaging and what to look for. Think of the mnemonic "ABCs": Adequacy and Alignment, Bones, Cartilages and Soft tissues.

- *Adequacy.* An adequate C-spine X-ray is one in which you can see the junction between the bodies of C7 and T1. If given a cervical spine X-ray in an exam and all you can see is C1–6, tell the examiners that this is not acceptable and you would like a further view. If they tell you that this is the best they could get and ask you what other methods you could use to improve the view, then say that you would like to repeat the X-ray with someone pulling down on the arms from the end of the bed or would like a swimmer's view (where the arm is abducted fully).
- *Alignment.* Assess four lines — the line that runs down the anterior vertebral bodies, the anterior vertebral canal, the posterior vertebral canal and the tips of the spinous processes. These should be curved with a slight lordosis. A step along this line or a loss of lordosis is abnormal (note whether the X-ray was taken with a hard collar on, because that can often be a cause for loss of lordosis). If the anteroposterior spinal canal space is narrowed, there is likely spinal cord compression.
- *Bones.* Look at the shape of the individual vertebral bodies (which should be rectangular), the lateral mass (the pedicles, facets, laminae and transverse processes) and the spinous processes.
- *Cartilages.* Assess the intervertebral discs (which should be of equal height) and facet joints.
- *Soft tissues.* Just anterior to the vertebral bodies are the soft tissues of the pharynx. If there is damage to the cervical spine, there is likely to be associated soft tissue swelling (haemorrhage). Look at the shadow of the prevertebral space for any swelling. In front of the upper cervical vertebrae its normal width is about half that of the vertebral body (or less than 5 mm). At about C4 the soft tissues take up more space with a width about equal to that of the vertebral body (as the larynx and oesophagus are here). If the space between the spinous processes is widened, this implies a torn interspinous ligament.

SHOCK

Shock is defined as an inadequate perfusion and tissue oxygenation of the vital organs (brain, heart, kidneys and skin). There are several causes of shock and they can be divided into haemorrhagic and non-haemorrhagic.

The non-haemorrhagic causes include cardiogenic, anaphylactic and septic shock (which should be known about but are not covered here). Tension pneumothorax is another cause of shock due to mediastinal shift and impairment of venous return.

Haemorrhagic Shock

Haemorrhage is the commonest cause of shock after injury. The most important step is to recognise and treat shock early even if the blood pressure is normal. As a rule any patient who is cool and tachycardic should be assumed to be shocked until proven otherwise.

The normal adult blood volume is 7% of body weight (about 5 l for a 70 kg man), whereas in a child it is about 9% of body weight, or 80 ml per kg. The body has excellent compensatory mechanisms to deal with volume loss (although as age increases these mechanisms become less efficient) and there may be no change in blood pressure until the loss is considerable.

On examination you should assess the appearance of the patient, the pulse, blood pressure, pulse pressure (the difference between the systolic and the diastolic blood pressure), respiratory rate, capillary refill time (normally less than 2 s), mental status and urine output.

There are four stages of shock based on the percentage of blood loss (Table 4.1). If you play tennis you will have no problem recalling the percentages, as the figures are the same as those used in the tennis scoring system.

Stage I Shock (0–15%)

This is up to 750 ml blood loss (based on a 70 kg man). This is the group that catches people out, as signs of shock are minimal. The patient is usually a little anxious; however, the pulse rate is usually less than 100 and the blood pressure and pulse pressure are normal.

Table 4.1.   Stages of Shock

	Stage I	Stage II	Stage III	Stage IV
Blood loss (%)	<15%	15–30%	30–40%	>40%
Blood loss (ml)	<750	750–1500	1500–2000	>2000
Consciousness	Slightly anxious	Agitated	Confused	Depressed
Pulse rate	<100	>100	>120	>140
Blood pressure	Normal	Normal	Decreased	Decreased
Pulse pressure	Normal	Decreased	Decreased	Decreased
Respiratory rate	14–20	20–30	30–40	>35
Urine output (ml/h)	>30	20–30	5–15	Negligible
Replacement	Crystalloid	Colloid	Colloid + blood	Colloid + blood

Stage II Shock (15–30%)

This is 750–1500 ml blood loss. Again the patient is anxious but the pulse is now above 100 and there is an increased respiratory rate. The systolic blood pressure is usually maintained (by vasoconstriction and increased cardiac output); however, the pulse pressure is now decreased, mainly because of a rise in the diastolic pressure.

Stage III Shock (30–40%)

This represents blood loss of up to 2000 ml. Now you see all the classic signs of inadequate perfusion, including marked tachycardia and tachyp-noea and a drop in the systolic blood pressure. There may be evidence of central nervous system impairment, such as confusion. It is therefore important to recognise shock in Stages I and II in order to prevent the patient from going into Stage III shock.

Stage IV Shock (Greater than 40%)

With a loss of greater than 2 l the condition is immediately life-threatening. The pulse is weak and thready, there is a significant drop in the systolic blood pressure (the diastolic blood pressure may be unrecordable), and the patient is pale, cold and clammy, with a depressed level of consciousness.

Management

Under C for "circulation", insert two large-bore cannulae (brown or grey), preferably one into each antecubital fossa. According to Poiseuille's law, flow is proportional to the fourth power of the internal radius of the tube and inversely proportional to the length, and so a short fat tube is essential. Note that a central line, although important for monitoring, is usually long and very thin and hence not effective for fluid resuscitation. If intravenous (IV) access is difficult in the antecubital fossae, then a femoral approach or a saphenous vein cut-down can be attempted (this is 2 cm above and anterior to the medial malleolus). In a child less than six years old, an interosseous needle can be used. This is a needle inserted directly into the tibia (just below the knee), allowing access to the vascular marrow, and can be used to replace blood and fluids in the same way as a venous cannula inserted into any other site.

Blood should be taken for laboratory analysis, including a cross-match, full blood count (FBC), U&E, glucose, toxicology studies and a pregnancy test in females of childbearing age. Blood gases are often useful at this stage. A central line (a catheter in a large central vein) may be inserted to help monitor fluid replacement or if cardiogenic shock is suspected.

Recent evidence has suggested that real-time ultrasound guidance for central line insertion, with or without Doppler assistance, improves catheter insertion success rates, reduces the number of venepuncture attempts prior to successful placement, and reduces the number of complications.

After fluid or blood administration, the response is monitored by the same signs and symptoms that are used to diagnose it. Urine output is the best indicator of the adequacy of resuscitation.

There are three types of response to the initial fluid resuscitation:

- *Rapid response*. Here the patients respond rapidly to the fluids and remain haemodynamically stable once the fluids are stopped or slowed. These patients have had minimal blood loss (< 20%) and can be observed but do not necessarily need any further intravenous fluids.

- *Transient response.* There is an initial response with a rise in the blood pressure and a fall in the pulse rate; however, as the fluids are slowed down, the indices used to measure shock start to deteriorate again, indicating that the blood loss is ongoing or resuscitation has been inadequate. The response to the fluid will indicate which patients are still slowly bleeding (as may other clinical findings).
- *No response.* This could be due to an exsanguinating haemorrhage and blood is needed rapidly. Type-specific blood (where the ABO and Rhesus groups are compatible, but there may be some minor antibodies that are incompatible) takes about 10 min to process and should be given initially in life-threatening bleeding whilst waiting for the full cross-match, which may take as long as 40 minutes. As a last resort, group O negative blood can be given, which is the universal donor.

Failure to respond to fluid resuscitation and blood indicates the need for immediate surgical intervention to control the haemorrhage ("turn off the tap"). Less commonly, a failure to respond may be due to the fact that there is a non-haemorrhagic cause for the shock, such as myocardial contusion or tamponade, and a CVP measurement may help to differentiate the causes.

If blood is given (usually packed red cells without plasma) it should be warmed to prevent hypothermia. After a large transfusion, platelets and fresh frozen plasma may be needed to correct the lack of clotting factors. The main aim of transfusion is to correct the oxygen-carrying capacity, since crystalloids and colloids can both correct the lack of intravascular volume but have no oxygen-carrying capacity.

Insertion of a Central Line

There are two main approaches: the first is known as the infraclavicular approach which inserts the central line into the subclavian vein, while the second approach inserts the central line into the internal jugular vein. A guide wire based on the Seldinger technique is employed.

In the infraclavicular approach, the patient is supine with the head down (about 15° as this helps to distend the neck veins and prevents an air embolism). The head should be supported by another helper if a cervical spine injury is suspected. An aseptic technique is used. Some local anaesthetic is infiltrated into the skin. A needle attached to a saline-filled syringe is introduced 1 cm below the junction of the middle and inner thirds of the clavicle. The needle is advanced medially and slightly upwards behind the clavicle (aiming for the sternal notch) as the plunger is slowly withdrawn. When venous blood enters the syringe, the syringe is removed, leaving the needle in the vein. A guide wire is inserted through the needle into the vein. The needle is removed, leaving the guide wire in the vein. The central line is then inserted over the guide wire and into the vein. The central line is fixed to the skin with a suture and is dressed. If necessary the central line is connected to a manometer to measure the central venous pressure (CVP).

The internal jugular approach is similar but via a different vein. The carotid pulse is felt just anterior to the midpoint of the sternocleidomastoid muscle (the high approach) and a needle is inserted lateral to this, aiming posteroinferiorly and towards the nipple on that side (the internal jugular vein lies posterior to the carotid artery at the base of the skull; the vein then twists around the carotid and lies lateral to it halfway down the neck and in front of it just below the clavicle).

In the low approach, the needle is inserted between the two heads of the sternocleidomastoid just above the clavicle.

After the central line has been inserted it is important to get a check X-ray to confirm the position of the line and rule out a pneumothorax.

Complications of central line insertion include the following:

- Pneumothorax and haemopneumothorax (especially in the subclavian approach)
- Arterial puncture (it is easier to apply pressure to the internal jugular if it is hit by mistake, than it is to the subclavian artery which is hidden deeply)
- Haematoma formation
- Infection

HEAD INJURIES

Introduction

Head injuries are common and range from a minor bump on the head that usually warrants simple advice but no investigation or treatment, through to the multiply injured patient with an associated head injury and a depressed level of consciousness. The majority of head injuries fall somewhere between these two extremes, and the difficulty for the doctor is in deciding who needs to be admitted for observation and who can be sent home. Questions on head injuries are common in finals.

Anatomy

The scalp has five layers, described by the mnemonic "SCALP": Skin, Connective tissue, Aponeurosis, Loose connective tissue and Periosteum (pericranium). It is highly vascular and can lead to large blood losses. Beneath the scalp is the skull, which contains the meninges, and then the brain. In a head injury any of these structures can be damaged.

Intracranial Pressure

The pressure within the skull is known as the intracranial pressure (ICP) and is actually the pressure which the subarachnoid space is under. Normally the ICP is less than 10 mmHg.

There is a simple yet vitally important concept relating to ICP dynamics, which is that the total volume of the intracranial contents must remain constant (known as the Monro–Kellie doctrine), which should be obvious since the skull in an adult is essentially a rigid structure that cannot expand.

The skull contains cerebrospinal fluid (CSF), blood and the brain. If the volume of one of these components increases, then the other two must decrease to compensate or the ICP will rise.

The ICP is usually maintained at a constant level by excellent autoregulatory mechanisms that can accommodate changes in the blood flow, so a normal ICP should not exclude a mass lesion.

We can accommodate a mass of about 50–100 ml without a significant rise in ICP. However, as the mass expands further, the autoregulatory

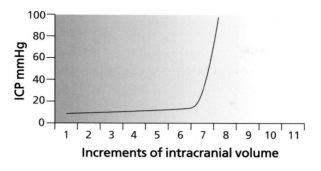

Figure 4.1. Graph of intracranial volume against intracranial pressure. Note that an expanding mass can initially be compensated as blood and CSF are squeezed out. However, the ICP rises rapidly after the period of compensation.

mechanisms fail and the rise in ICP is rapid (as is the patient's deterioration) and can lead to brain herniation (Figure 4.1).

Cerebral Perfusion Pressure (CPP)

The cerebral perfusion pressure is just as important as the ICP as it is a measure of the amount of oxygenated blood reaching the brain:

$$CPP = \text{Mean arterial BP} - ICP.$$

Large increases in the ICP lead to a decrease in the cerebral perfusion pressure.

As the CPP falls there is initially electrical followed by structural brain damage, and a prolonged CPP of less than 70 mmHg is usually associated with a poor outcome following head injury.

Cerebral blood flow is dependent on both the arterial PCO_2 and the systemic blood pressure. As the arterial PCO_2 rises cerebrovasodilatation occurs, worsening the raised ICP. In reverse, reducing the arterial PCO_2 reduces the cerebral blood volume and hence the intracranial pressure. Therefore, in cases of a raised ICP the patient should be hyperventilated to keep the PCO_2 low.

Maintenance of the CPP is one of the priorities of management of a patient with a severe head injury.

Types of Injury

Scalp Laceration

Lacerations of the scalp can bleed profusely and lead to major blood loss, especially in children.

Skull Fracture

Skull fractures are common. It is possible to have one without severe brain injury, and likewise you can have an intracranial injury without an accompanying skull fracture, especially in children, whose bones and joints are more supple. The only significance of X-raying head injury patients and looking for a skull fracture is that such patients have a statistically higher probability of developing a bleed into the brain, and hence they get admitted for observation. The types of fracture are as follows:

- *Linear (non-depressed) fracture*. This appears as a lucent line.
- *Depressed skull fracture*. Management will depend on the underlying brain injury. The fragment may need to be elevated if depressed more than the thickness of the skull or if there are focal signs.
- *Open skull fracture*. This usually requires operative intervention. A broad-spectrum antibiotic should be started, the patient taken to theatre for wound debridement and the fracture dealt with.
- *Basal skull fracture*. This fracture cannot usually be seen on a plain X-ray of the skull, although it should be suspected if there are fluid levels in the sphenoidal sinuses. The diagnosis is made on clinical findings of the CSF leaking from the nose (rhinorrhoea) or the ears (otorrhoea). The CSF is usually crystal clear, unless it is bloodstained. It can be tested for by allowing a drop to fall onto a piece of filter paper. The blood remains at the centre and the CSF soaks around it in concentric rings of clear fluid, called the halo sign. Other clinical signs of a basal skull fracture include the battle sign (bruising around the mastoid region due to tracking of blood under the skin) and haemotympanum (blood behind the tympanic membrane), which together with CSF otorrhoea are indicative of a middle fossa fracture

through the petrous temporal bone. The badger sign (bruising around both orbits), together with rhinorrhoea, is associated with a fracture of the cribriform plate. The badger and battle signs may, however, take several hours to develop.

Brain Injury

Injuries to the brain can be primary, occurring at the time of impact; or secondary to hypovolaemia, hypoxia, hypoglycaemia and raised intracranial pressure. Prevention of primary brain injury can only be brought about by measures to stop the accident from happening in the first place, such as having road speed limits and wearing motorcycle helmets. The main aim in the management of a head injury is, therefore, to prevent or limit the damage that occurs due to secondary injury.

Primary brain damage can be diffuse or focal.

Diffuse Injuries

- *Concussion.* This is a brain injury accompanied by a temporary loss of neurological function. The changes are reversible and are often resolved by the time the patient arrives at the hospital. They may have just been confused or dazed at the scene or may have lost consciousness. Afterwards they may complain of a headache, feel dizzy, be amnesic or nauseous, and generally if the patient has been unconscious for more than five minutes it is probably best to admit them to hospital for observation.
- *Diffuse axonal injury.* This is a more severe injury, with microscopic structural damage throughout the brain tissue. It is often characterised by prolonged coma and can last from days to weeks. Such patients can develop autonomic dysfunction and hence have high fevers, hypertension and sweating. The mortality is high.

Focal Injuries

- *Contusions.* These are focal areas of brain injury. They can be *coup* injuries, where the brain is damaged directly by the skull at the point of impact; or *contre coup* injuries, where the brain is squashed by the skull at a remote point from the impact.

The patient may have a focal neurological deficit, depending on the site of the contusion. Oedema may develop at the site of damage and cause neurological deterioration. The patient is usually managed conservatively; however, due to the risk of delayed bleeding into the contusion, careful observation for deterioration is needed (especially in alcoholics).

Intracranial haemorrhage. This can be meningeal or into the brain tissue.

○ *Acute extradural/epidural haemorrhage.* This is due to a bleed from the arteries that supply the skull and dura — usually the middle meningeal artery, which sits just under the skull in a region called the pterion (or temple). This type of bleed is quite rare, accounting for less than 1% of coma-producing head injuries; however, it can be rapidly fatal. There is usually an associated skull fracture of the parietal or temporal bone, often caused by a direct blow, for example, being hit over the side of the head by a baseball bat.

The typical picture is loss of consciousness (concussion), followed by a lucid interval. During this lucid interval the haematoma is expanding into the extradural space and compressing the brain inwards, stripping the dura off the skull as it expands (hence the convex appearance of the clot on the CT). As mentioned before, the ICP does not rise initially as the mass is accommodated; however, once the clot reaches a critical volume the ICP increases rapidly.

The rapid rise in the ICP causes a secondary lapse in the level of consciousness. As the ICP rises further the uncus (the medial aspect of the temporal lobe) herniates through the tentorium (the layer that divides the cerebral hemispheres from the brain stem and cerebellum). The third nerve passes through this opening and can be compressed at this point. The patient initially develops a constriction of the pupil on the affected side, which then begins to dilate (Hutchinson's pupil). The fixed dilated pupil on the affected side is usually accompanied by a hemiparesis on the opposite side (remember the corticospinal fibres cross over). As the pressure continues to increase, the opposite pupil dilates and eventually the brain stem "cones" through the foramen magnum.

This injury requires immediate surgical intervention. The patient should have a CT as early as possible if this type of injury is suspected. Neurosurgical advice should be sought and the patient transferred if necessary for surgical evacuation of the clot. If the injury is treated early the prognosis is excellent.

o *Acute subdural haemorrhage.* This is much more common than an extradural haemorrhage, and occurs in about 30% of severe head injuries. It is usually due to rupture of a bridging vein between the cerebral cortex and the dura (but it can also be due to laceration of the cerebral cortex), and is often caused by a rotational injury. The elderly are more susceptible, as their brains are often shrunken and hence the bridging veins are put under tension. The bleeding is typically less brisk than an extradural haemorrhage, but clinically it can present with symptoms of an expanding mass as in the previous type of haemorrhage. The prognosis is much worse and the mortality high.

o *Subarachnoid haemorrhage.* This can be associated with trauma, although it is usually due to hypertension and bleeding from berry aneurysms. The symptoms are those of meningeal irritation similar to meningitis.

o *Brain haemorrhages and lacerations.* These are tears to the brain substance with bleeding into them. The deficit will depend on the site of the damage. These injuries are therefore similar to strokes, and surgery cannot help the patient. Rehabilitation can be very slow.

Assessment of Severe Head Injuries

As the patient is brought into casualty you should attempt to get some history, finding out as much as possible about the incident. If they are unconscious the history is taken from witnesses or the ambulance crew. Perform the primary survey according to ATLS® guidelines — ABCDE.

The Glasgow Coma Scale is a quantitative measure of the patient's level of consciousness. It is divided into three parts: assessing the best motor response, the best eye opening response and the best verbal

Table 4.2.   Glasgow Coma Scale

	Score
Best Eye Opening	
Spontaneous	4
To voice	3
To pain	2
None	1
Best Verbal Response	
Oriented	5
Confused	4
Inappropriate speech	3
Incomprehensible speech	2
No speech	1
Best Motor Response	
Obeys commands	6
Localises to pain	5
Withdraws from pain	4
Flexes to pain	3
Extends to pain	2
None	1
Total	3–15

response. It was devised to allow comparisons to be made (if necessary by different observers) to see if the patient's consciousness has improved or deteriorated. The minimum score is 3 and the maximum 15 (Table 4.2).

A GCS score of 8 or less implies coma and a severe head injury. If the score is greater than 8, then the patient is not in a coma. A GCS score of 9–12 implies a moderate head injury and a GCS score of 13–15 indicates a minor head injury.

The vital signs and the GCS should be repeated at regular intervals, and deterioration by more than two points should be taken very seriously and a neurosurgical consultation sought. Remember that although bleeding from a scalp wound can cause shock, bleeding into the skull cannot. Therefore never assume that hypotension is due to an intracranial bleed or to brain injury (as this is a terminal event on failure of the medullary centres). Look for another cause.

The Cushing response is a combination of progressive hypertension, bradycardia and a decreased respiratory rate (the opposite of hypo-volaemic shock). It is due to a lethal rise in the ICP, usually because of an intracranial bleed needing urgent decompression. Hypertension alone or with hyperthermia suggests central autonomic dysfunction caused by dif-fuse brain injury.

Under D for "disability", document the patient's level of conscious-ness using the AVPU score. If the airway, breathing and circulation are under control, then the mini-neurological examination can be performed in the primary survey; otherwise it is performed in the secondary survey.

The mini-neurological examination involves three components:

- *Level of consciousness.* The Glasgow Coma Scale.
- *Pupillary function.* Are the pupils equal and reactive to light?
- *Lateralising neurology.* Swiftly assess the tone, power and reflexes of all four limbs.

The purpose of this is to detect those with a severe head injury who are likely to need surgery (i.e. those with abnormalities of all three components).

Remember that the initial neurological examination is only a baseline for comparing the results of repeated examinations, in order to determine deterioration or improvement of the patient's condition.

Management of Severe Head Injuries

This involves, first, dealing with the life-threatening injuries (ABC); then, assessing the severity of the head injury, whilst preventing secondary brain damage from occurring, by ensuring optimal cerebral metabolic supplies and preventing intracranial hypertension.

Cerebral Metabolism

The brain requires oxygen and glucose to function, so adequate substrates must be present in the circulation to meet this requirement. The oxygen content depends on both the arterial haemoglobin and the PO_2.

The PO_2 can be measured by blood gases, and oxygen can be supplemented as necessary. If the haemoglobin is low a transfusion may be required to improve the oxygen-carrying capacity.

Raised Intracranial Pressure

This may be due to a mass lesion or brain oedema, and should be treated.

In cases of raised ICP the patient should be hyperventilated to keep the PCO_2 low (see section on ICP). To do this it is usually necessary to intubate and ventilate the patient, so early involvement of an anaesthetist is essential. Remember that a decrease in the PCO_2 leads to a decrease in the cerebral blood flow and so the PCO_2 must be kept at about 3.5 as a compromise.

Intravenous fluids may be needed in the management of other problems, such as shock, and the risk is that overhydration may make cerebral oedema worse. Therefore, isotonic fluids such as Hartmann's solution should be administered, rather than hypo-osmolar fluids such as dextrose.

Diuretics such as mannitol are often used to reduce intracranial pressure, and are given if a mass lesion is suspected whilst awaiting transfer to a neurosurgical unit, although a neurosurgical consultation should be obtained prior to giving any diuretics. (If diuretics are used a urinary catheter is required to aid fluid balance measurement.) Steroids have no place in the acute management of head injuries.

Management of Mild to Moderate Head Injuries

The problem for a casualty officer when they see what appears to be a minor head injury is in deciding who needs admitting for observation. In general the history is very important.

Falls from a height should be taken very seriously, as they have a much greater risk of an intracranial bleed than road traffic accidents. For a fall, inquire about the height of the fall and whether it was onto concrete or grass, etc. If the patient was driving a car, inquire about the speed of the car and whether a seat-belt was worn, whether any of the other passengers were injured or killed, and whether alcohol or drugs were involved. Was consciousness lost and if so for how long? Has the patient regained consciousness since the accident or have they remained unconscious ever since? Has the patient fitted since or complained of visual disturbances, dizziness or a worsening headache?

Document the amnesia for the events that led up to the incident (retrograde amnesia) or for the events that followed the incident (anterograde amnesia). The length of anterograde amnesia has been shown to be a good indicator of the severity of the head injury (less than 1 h — mild; 1–24 h — moderate; more than 24 h — severe), although this is not much help in the initial assessment, which takes place soon after the incident. With children it is also worth noting whether they cried immediately, as this is a good sign (i.e. normal behaviour), or whether they were limp and unresponsive.

Examination is essentially the same as above; however, in some cases it is difficult to decide what investigations are needed and whether or not you can safely send the patient home. For example, let us say the patient has walked into the department after a head injury sustained in an assault where they were hit over the head with a brick. Speech is slurred from drink and there is a bump on the forehead, but no focal neurologic signs are found on examination (within the limits of the cooperation of this patient).

A large proportion of patients present like this. Should you X-ray these patients?

X-rays may help in deciding who should be admitted for observation, but not much else. Statistically if there is a skull fracture, then the risk of an intracranial bleed is significantly higher (Table 4.3).

Indications for performing an X-ray include the following (but do check the protocol at your hospital):

- Loss of consciousness for more than a few minutes
- Neurological symptoms or signs (unless a CT is indicated) such as visual disturbances, dizziness, weakness, persistent vomiting

Table 4.3. Rough Risk of Intracranial Haematoma in Adults

	No skull fracture	Skull fracture
Fully conscious	<1/1000	1/30
Depressed consciousness	1/100	1/4

- Signs of a basal skull fracture
- Suspected penetrating injuries (X-rays are essential in this case)
- Common sense, i.e. history of significant injury or obvious significant scalp wound
- When there is difficulty in assessing the patient (young/old, drunk, postepileptic)

The indications for admission are as follows:

- Skull fracture
- Depressed level of consciousness or confusion when examined
- Neurological symptoms or signs
- Difficult to assess
- Social circumstances (e.g. patient lives alone, with no responsible adult to observe them)

If the patient is admitted, they are usually given non-opiate analgesia (or codeine phosphate, which is safe to use) and taken to the ward. Regular neurological observations are performed, initially on an hourly basis.

The observations include vital signs, GCS, pupils and motor function, and are represented schematically on a graph to detect any deterioration.

If the patient is not admitted they should be sent home with head injury instructions (go to your casualty department and get a copy) accompanied by a responsible adult who will bring them back should their condition deteriorate.

BURNS

Different types of burns tend to affect different age groups. Toddlers tend to be scalded, for example, by pulling the kettle wire or the pan off the stove, children tend to set their clothes on fire, while the old tend to suffer domestic accidents at home. The majority of adult burns, however, are associated with industrial accidents (or are drug- or alcohol-related).

Pathology

The damage is caused by coagulation of proteins with cell death. The burn can affect any depth of skin. The superficial burn causes vasodilatation with diffuse erythema, where kinins are released and pain is felt. As the depth increases, the capillaries become damaged and therefore more permeable, leading to blistering and oedema formation. As the dermis becomes involved, the nerve endings which lie here are damaged and sensation is lost. Once the germinal layer is damaged, the skin will never regrow, and these burns heal with fibrosis and contractures. The damaged necrotic tissue lying in a protein-rich exudate is an ideal medium for infection. The increased capillary permeability can lead to the exudation of protein-rich fluid from the surface of the burn and oedema into the surrounding tissues. The patient can very quickly become hypovolaemic.

Types of Burns

- Thermal — dry (fire) or wet (hot liquids and gases)
- Chemical
- Electrical
- Friction

Chemical burns result from exposure to acids, alkalis or petroleum products. In general, alkali burns are more serious than acid burns as they penetrate more deeply. The chemical should be flushed away from the skin with copious amounts of irrigation with water (20–30 min). If dry powder is present, brush it away before irrigating. Neutralising agents are no better than water.

Electrical burns are more serious than they appear. The overlying skin may look normal, but deeper tissue may be damaged. Rhabdomyolysis leads to myoglobin release and the risk of acute renal failure. The patient can also develop cardiac disturbance due to acidosis and changes in potassium concentration. A cardiac monitor and a urinary catheter are therefore necessary. The patient will have dark urine due to the myoglobin and require large amounts of fluids to ensure a high urine output. If necessary, mannitol can be used to maintain diuresis and flush out the myoglobin.

Management of the Burns Patient

The management of the burns patient, as with any trauma patient, is to exclude any life-threatening injuries first (i.e. ABCDE, according to

ATLS® guidelines). The main priorities with burns patients, however, are as follows:

- Securing the airway
- Management of fluid loss
- Prevention of infection

Immediate Resuscitation

Secure the airway, and stop the burning process by removing all clothing.

Airway

The supraglottic airway can rapidly become obstructed due to oedema and swelling following a burn injury. It is therefore important to suspect involvement of the airway, even if the patient is breathing normally when first examined. Apart from the obvious signs of airway injury, such as stridor or hoarseness, any of the following should alert the doctor to the likely presence of an acute inhalation injury:

- Facial burns
- Singeing of the eyebrows or nasal hairs
- Carbonaceous sputum
- Altered consciousness
- History — such as long exposure to smoke or gases, or an explosion

An anaesthetist must be called immediately. Early endotracheal intubation is better than adopting a wait-and-see policy, as the airway can become obstructed rapidly.

Breathing

Apart from direct thermal injury, which causes upper airway oedema and obstruction, inhalation of toxic fumes and smoke can lead to chemical tracheobronchitis, oedema and pneumonia. You should always assume carbon monoxide (CO) exposure if the patient was confined to an enclosed area.

CO has an affinity for haemoglobin that is about 240 times that of oxygen, and hence oxygen is displaced and the oxygen dissociation curve is shifted to the left. The CO dissociates very slowly when the patient is breathing room air (with a half-life of about 6 h). If 100% oxygen is breathed the half-life is shortened to about 40 min. Therefore, the patient should have arterial blood gases taken for assessment of the carboxyhaemoglobin concentration and 100% oxygen should be commenced. Symptoms may include headache, nausea, vomiting or confusion at high levels of exposure, but the classic cherry-red skin appearance is rare.

Circulation

It may be difficult to get a reliable blood pressure owing to the burns, so the urine output is probably the best indicator of circulating blood volume.

Establish intravenous access if necessary through the burnt skin, and start 2 l of Hartmann's solution immediately. The fluid losses can be huge and a 50% burns patient can lose up to half their plasma volume in about 3–4 h.

A rough guide is to replace 2–4 ml of crystalloid fluid for each kilogram body weight per percentage burn in the first 24 h. So a 70 kg man with a 50% burn will require 7–14 l in the first 24 h ($2 \times 70 \times 50 = 7000$ ml $= 7$ l). Half the fluid should be given in the first 8 h from the time of the burn (not the time of arrival to casualty), so if the burn was 2 h before arrival, the patient will need at the very minimum 3.5 l of fluids in the next 6 h.

In some departments the policy is to replace colloids such as human albumin solution (HAS), and in this case the Muir and Barclay formula can be used. This determines how much plasma volume is needed in terms of colloid replacement.

Volume of colloid needed (per unit time) = weight (kg) × percentage burn/2.

So, for a 70 kg man with a 50% burn this would be 1.75 l of colloid per unit time ($70 \times 50/2 = 1750$ ml). The first amount is given in the first 4 h from the burn, then the same amount in the subsequent 4 h, 4 h, 6 h, 6 h and 12 h. This would total about 8.75 l of colloid in the first day and in addition crystalloid maintenance (about 3 l) with, say, normal saline is required.

Remember that these figures are just guides and no matter whether crystalloids or colloids have been administered, the best indicator of sufficient replacement is an adequate urine output of greater than 30–50 ml/h. The haematocrit is also used to guide fluid balance.

Circumferential full-thickness burns can impede the blood supply to the limbs owing to oedema in a confined space (a tourniquet effect), and are best treated by escharotomies (incisions through scar tissue). The incision is made along the line of the limb through the entire scar. As this is a full-thickness burn, sensation is absent and in theory no anaesthetic is required. In practice, however, the escharotomy tends to be done with the patient anaesthetised (because there are some areas of partial-thickness burns adjacent to the full-thickness zones which will clearly cause pain). Cross-matched blood must be available, as this procedure can cause profuse bleeding. Circumferential burns of the thorax may cause restriction of chest expansion, and bilateral escharotomies may be needed to improve breathing.

Assessing the Burn (History, Size and Depth of the Burn)

History

Note the cause and exact time of the burn (remember to ask about associated injuries, for example, whether the patient jumped out of a window to escape the fire). Try to ascertain some past medical history, such as diabetes, hypertension, heart or lung disease, the medication the patient is on, allergies and tetanus status.

Depth of Burn

Superficial burns (also called first-degree burns) are not life-threatening and are simply painful red areas, such as sunburn. There is no blistering and in the long term they usually do not scar.

In partial-thickness burns (also called deep dermal or second-degree burns) there is associated swelling and blistering, and the skin is red and may be oozing fluid. These burns are very painful and sensitive even to air currents. In the long term, most deep dermal burns do not scar but it very much depends on the patient's skin type and whether or not they need a skin graft (for example, there have been cases of marked keloid scarring following a deep dermal burn in black patients even without surgery).

In full-thickness burns (also called third-degree burns) the skin is dry, painless and insensate; it may appear pale, white or charred. In the long term these will scar.

Body Surface Area (BSA)

The "rule of nines" is a useful way to determine the extent of the burn. The adult body is divided into regions that represent 9% of the body area, except for the genital region which is considered to be 1% of the BSA (Figure 4.2). The proportions are different in children as the head contributes more than the legs to the total area (as it does for heat loss). Another good guide is that the patient's palm (not your palm and not including the patient's fingers) represents about 1% of the body surface area.

You can use these guides to estimate that in an adult with a burn to one arm and one leg with a small area affected on the torso of about three palm sizes, the percentage burn is about 30% (9 + 18 + 3).

Summary of Management of the Burns Patient

- Airway: Look for signs of obstruction or signs indicating the risk of obstruction; inform the anaesthetist
- Breathing: Pulse oximetry; look for signs of CO poisoning, 100% oxygen, arterial blood gas analysis; request a chest X-ray
- Circulation: IV access × 2. Take blood for FBC, U&E, glucose, cross-match and carboxyhaemoglobin levels. Start IV fluids, ECG; catheterise if necessary
- Assess the burn depth and body surface area, adjust fluid requirements, consider escharotomies
- Analgesia: This usually involves opiates, titrated to the patient's pain
- Assess for associated injuries; a nasogastric tube may be needed

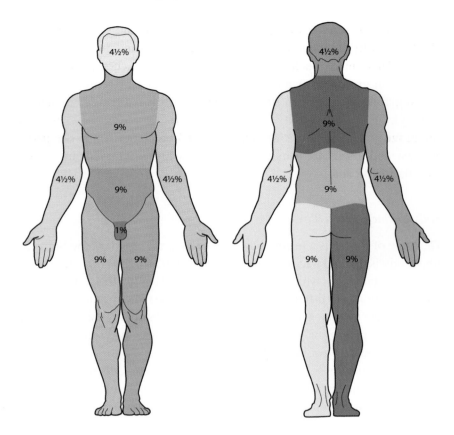

Figure 4.2.   The "rule of nines".

- Cover the burns as partial-thickness burns are painful even when in contact with air currents; gently cover them with sterile towels. Do not apply any antiseptic and do not pierce the blisters
- Take extra special precautions to avoid infection, which after the initial resuscitation is the main cause of morbidity and mortality. The patient should be transferred to a regional burns unit if necessary, especially if:

    o   There is a partial-thickness burn of greater than 20% BSA (in the very young or old a 10% burn should be referred)
    o   Full-thickness burn of greater than 5%

○ Involvement of the face, hands, feet, genitalia or over major joints
○ Significant chemical or electrical burns
○ There is an inhalation injury or other serious comorbidity

The burns should be covered with cling film, then have warm blankets applied before transfer as the use of agents such as sulphasalizine or paraffin gauze interfere with the assessment of the burn when the patient arrives at the burns unit.

5

LIVER, BILIARY TRACT AND PANCREAS

Richard Charnley

Many of the pathological entities in this section appear in both medicine and surgery, and questions on them may therefore be found in either part of the examination. There is, however, often a difference in emphasis between the types of answer one should give in a medical examination and in a surgical examination, even when dealing with the same condition. Having said that, most surgeons work closely with their physician colleagues and, despite differences in emphasis, they will usually have similar views about management and the precise role of surgical intervention.

INVESTIGATIONS

The relevant investigations for most conditions of the liver, biliary tract and pancreas are blood tests (including liver function tests) and diagnostic imaging.

Liver Function Tests (LFTs)

The usual liver function tests are listed in Table 5.1.

In addition, the prothrombin time or INR (the international ratio, i.e. the length of time the patient's blood takes to clot in comparison with a normal person's blood) may be abnormal and should be checked in any jaundiced patient or when defective liver synthesis is suspected. If abnormal it can be corrected by vitamin K (which is a fat-soluble

Table 5.1.   Liver Function Tests

Bilirubin	A rise in bilirubin is the definition of "jaundice". It is bilirubin which makes the patient yellow.
Alkaline phosphatase	This enzyme tends to be raised more with obstruction of the bile ducts (i.e. obstructive jaundice).
Transaminases (e.g. ALT, AST)	These tend to be raised more with defective liver cell function (i.e. hepatocellular dysfunction).
Albumin	This is synthesised by the liver and is therefore low in patients with chronic liver disease and malnutrition.
Gamma GT	This enzyme is raised in both hepatocellular and obstructive disorders.

vitamin and is not absorbed well in many forms of liver disease because of a lack of bile salts, which are required to emulsify fats in the intestinal lumen).

IMAGING TECHNIQUES

Ultrasound (Transabdominal)

This is non-invasive and is the first imaging investigation of choice in patients with hepatobiliary or pancreatic disease.

Computed Tomography (CT)

CT of the liver and pancreas, particularly if carried out on a multislice scanner, provides good views of the organs of the upper abdomen. It is very useful in diagnosing and staging suspected tumours and is also of importance in identifying the degree of severity in acute pancreatitis and complications in chronic pancreatitis.

Magnetic Resonance Imaging (MRI)

MRI is of value in imaging the bile duct and pancreatic duct (known as magnetic resonance cholangiopancreatography or MRCP). MRI of the liver is commonly used for the assessment of malignant tumours.

Endoscopic Ultrasound (EUS)

With an ultrasound transducer on the end of an endoscope, EUS provides good images of the gallbladder, bile duct and pancreas. It is useful for identifying bile duct stones and gallbladder microlithiasis; detecting and staging pancreatobiliary tumours; assessing pancreatic cystic lesions; identifying early parenchymal and ductal changes in chronic pancreatitis; and screening for pancreatic cancer. It is also safer than ERCP, particularly with regard to the risk of postprocedure pancreatitis. Fine-needle aspiration (FNA) under EUS guidance is a valuable method of obtaining positive cytology in pancreatic cancer.

Endoscopic Retrograde Cholangiopancreatography (ERCP)

A side-viewing endoscope is passed into the duodenum and then the bile duct or pancreatic duct is cannulated. In addition, endoscopic sphincterotomy and stone extraction can be carried out for biliary stones or a biliary or pancreatic stent can be inserted for relief of obstruction. The complications of ERCP can be serious and include acute pancreatitis, bleeding, perforation and cholangitis. These complications can be reduced by investigating patients with endoscopic ultrasound or MRCP and by reserving ERCP for those patients who are likely to require a therapeutic procedure.

Percutaneous Transhepatic Cholangiography (PTC)

This procedure provides percutaneous access to the biliary tract and is mainly used in those patients with a hilar obstruction or in those where ERCP has failed to relieve the biliary obstruction.

Liver Biopsy and Pancreatic Biopsy

If a patient has a liver tumour or pancreatic tumour which is suspicious of malignancy, percutaneous biopsy carries a risk of causing peritoneal metastasis and is only used if resectional surgery is not contemplated. Liver biopsy is usually used for parenchymal disorders such as cirrhosis. Pancreatic biopsy may be carried out at the time of endo-scopic ultrasound.

GALLSTONES

Gallstones are very common and are therefore frequently asked about in finals. The majority are asymptomatic and require no treatment. They can, however, cause a wide range of clinical problems, depending on their posi-tion. They are either made up of cholesterol or pigment (composed of bilirubin breakdown products) or a mixture of the two. Pure pigment stones are rare (<10%) and are found in conditions such as haemolytic anaemia. Most (75%) gallstones are predominantly cholesterol. Ninety percent of gallstones are radiolucent, i.e. they do not show up on a plain X-ray (unlike renal calculi, of which 90% are radio-opaque). Predisposing factors to gall-stone formation include female sex (three times more common), obesity, age (10% of those over 50 years old have gallstones, and 30% of those over 70 years old have gallstones), haemolytic anaemia, hyperlipidaemias and Crohn's disease. Some people also appear to have an innate tendency to form gallstones and are said to have lithogenic bile. People often refer to the typical gallstone patient as fat, female, fertile and 40.

The complications of gallstones are as follows:

- In the gallbladder
  - Chronic cholecystitis
  - Biliary colic
  - Acute cholecystitis
    - Empyema
    - Biliary peritonitis
    - Abscess
  - Mucocele
  - Carcinoma of gallbladder
- In the common bile duct
  - Obstructive jaundice
  - Cholangitis
  - Acute pancreatitis
- In the gut
  - Gallstone ileus

CHRONIC CHOLECYSTITIS

Chronic cholecystitis is a term used to describe symptoms of upper abdominal pain, indigestion, bloating, burping, nausea and occasional vomiting. Sometimes this symptom complex is called flatulent dyspepsia. The patient may describe the symptoms as being precipitated by fatty food (fats stimulate the release of cholecystokinin, which causes gallbladder contractions). There is usually nothing to find on physical examination. The main differential diagnoses include peptic ulceration, hiatus hernia and irritable bowel syndrome. Because gallstones are common it is important not to automatically ascribe such symptoms to them simply because gallstones are present on an ultrasound scan. A missed peptic ulcer or irritable bowel syndrome will obviously not be helped by unnecessary cholecystectomy and the patient will continue to get symptoms (sometimes called postcholecystectomy syndrome). If the symptoms are thought to be arising from the gallbladder and are significant, then the treatment is cholecystectomy, usually laparoscopic. Attempts to dissolve gallstones using bile salt therapy are possible only in patients with small, non-calcified stones and are reserved for those who refuse or are unfit for surgery. This treatment is not very successful.

BILIARY COLIC

Biliary colic is the pain caused by the gallbladder contracting against a stone stuck in the neck of the gallbladder (Hartmann's pouch) or the cystic duct. It may account for some of the symptoms of chronic cholecystitis. Unlike intestinal colic, the pain is continuous and not in waves. It is usually felt in the epigastrium or right upper quadrant and may radiate around both costal margins and into the back. The pain can be extremely severe and patients may be sweaty, pale and tachycardic because of it. They may also feel nauseated or vomit. They will usually be unable to get comfortable and will prefer to writhe around rather than stay still. Attacks usually last less than 6 h and examination is usually otherwise normal. Differential diagnoses include other causes of severe upper abdominal pain, such as perforated peptic ulcer, pancreatitis or ruptured aneurysm. Management involves giving analgesia, investigation to confirm gallstones (ultrasound) and subsequent elective cholecystectomy in most cases.

ACUTE CHOLECYSTITIS

In its earliest stage this may appear to be biliary colic, and indeed many attacks of acute cholecystitis probably start with biliary colic. Most episodes of acute cholecystitis are caused by chemical inflammation within an obstructed gallbladder and the exact mechanisms are poorly understood. Bacterial infection probably is a secondary event in about one third of cases and these may be the ones most likely to develop complications. Patients will typically have severe right upper quadrant or epigastric pain. Like biliary colic, this may radiate around the costal margins or into the back. Unlike biliary colic, patients will prefer to lie still and take shallow breaths (this is now a form of local peritonitis, not colic). They will usually have a temperature and tachycardia, and may also have nausea and vomiting. Murphy's sign may be positive. This is often asked about in vivas. It is elicited by pressing in the right upper quadrant under the costal margin. The patient is then asked to breathe in, and winces or gasps with pain as the gallbladder moves down and hits the examiner's hand. The test should also be performed in the left upper quadrant to exclude non-specific reactions due to other pathology.

A mass may be present in the right upper quadrant, but if so this is not usually the gallbladder itself but rather phlegmon (i.e. inflamed and adherent omentum and bowel around the gallbladder).

The treatment of acute cholecystitis is initial resuscitation with intravenous fluids and antibiotics. The patient will normally be kept nil by mouth or on sips of clear fluids, and initial investigations will be arranged, including basic blood tests such as full blood count (FBC) (usually the white cell count is raised), urea and electrolytes (U&E), LFTs and amylase (as acute pancreatitis may be a differential diagnosis). The most important confirmatory test is usually an ultrasound scan. This can confirm gallstones, show thickening and oedema of the gallbladder wall and localise the tender spot to the gallbladder itself. It can also exclude dilatation of the common bile duct and other pathology, such as liver masses. Only very occasionally is a HIDA scan used to help confirm or exclude cholecystitis. The principle of this test is that HIDA (a radioisotope) is taken up by the liver and excreted into the bile. If the cystic duct is patent it will fill the gallbladder effectively, excluding cholecystitis.

With conservative treatment approximately 80–90% of cases of acute cholecystitis will settle over the next 24–48 h (i.e. the pain settles, the temperature falls and the patient's abdomen becomes non-tender). In about 10% there will not be a prompt resolution of symptoms and signs, and in these cases surgery is usually advised. Particularly worrying signs are increasing temperature, tachycardia and the onset of increasing tenderness or signs of peritonitis. These may indicate infarction of the gallbladder (gangrenous cholecystitis) or perforation, which may produce either a local collection or generalised peritonitis. A gallbladder full of pus (empyema of the gallbladder) usually leads to an unwell patient with signs of sepsis (e.g. fever, tachycardia, hypotension) as well as pain and tenderness in the right upper quadrant.

More controversial is the question of what to do with patients who do not absolutely require early surgery. Although conventional management is to allow the acute episode to settle down and to readmit the patient for elective cholecystectomy six to eight weeks later, many surgeons now prefer laparoscopic cholecystectomy in the acute phase. This allows patients to recover more quickly and to be spared further episodes of pain.

CHOLECYSTECTOMY

Laparoscopic cholecystectomy has now replaced open cholecystectomy in the majority of cases. Open cholecystectomy may still be indicated in difficult cases or when laparoscopic cholecystectomy has been attempted and has failed. The open operation is usually performed through a right subcostal incision or occasionally through an upper midline. The gallbladder is dissected off the liver. The cystic artery and cystic duct are then identified, ligated and divided (note: there is no cystic vein). Great care should be taken not to damage the bile duct.

The first laparoscopic cholecystectomy was performed in 1987 by Phillipe Mouret (a gynaecologist!) in France and the procedure has since become accepted as the mainstay treatment of uncomplicated gallstone disease. Laparoscopy (peritoneoscopy) involves insertion of a rigid endoscope into the peritoneal cavity, which is insufflated with carbon dioxide gas, to provide a view of the abdominal contents. The advantages of minimal access surgery are attributable to the smaller wounds used for the laparoscopic ports. This results in less postoperative pain, less chance of wound infection, reduced postoperative chest complications and earlier mobilisation and discharge from hospital as well as earlier return to work. The main disadvantage of laparoscopic surgery is the loss of tactile feedback and the potential for tumour implantation if an incidental carcinoma of the gallbladder is present. The only current contraindications to laparoscopic cholecystectomy are suspected cancer and patients with bleeding disorders or portal hypertension. Multiple adhesions may make laparoscopy difficult.

You do not need to know how to carry out operations for finals; however, it is worth knowing the principles of key operations, at the very least.

Laparoscopic Cholecystectomy Procedure

Access to the peritoneal cavity is achieved at the umbilicus by direct exposure of the peritoneum and insertion of a blunt trochar. The pneumoperitoneum is created by insufflation of carbon dioxide. The intra-abdominal pressure is kept at about 15 mmHg, just enough to keep the anterior abdominal wall off the viscera. The camera is introduced through the umbilical port and three further ports are sited under direct vision, one in the epigastrium, one at the right costal margin and one in the right flank, to allow the instruments and graspers access.

The gallbladder is retracted upwards, lifting the liver and allowing the whole gallbladder to be visualised. The position of the patient (head-up tilt and rotation to the left by 15–20°) improves visualisation. The neck of the gallbladder is dissected off the liver by incising the peritoneum anteriorly and posteriorly. This allows a window to be created between the liver and neck of the gallbladder. The cystic artery and cystic duct are then identified. It is mandatory to confirm that the right hepatic artery is not mistaken for the cystic artery. This artery must be shown to be passing only to the gallbladder. The cystic duct is then identified joining the gallbladder. Creation of the large window between the neck of the gallbladder and the liver is essential to avoid bile duct injury. If an operative cholangiogram is to be performed, a cannula is inserted into the cystic duct and retained with a clip whilst the cholangiogram is carried out (dye is injected under an image intensifier). If the cholangiogram is satisfactory (normal anatomy, no bile duct stones and flow of contrast into the duodenum), the cannula is withdrawn and the cystic duct clipped and divided above two clips. The gallbladder is then dissected off the liver and removed through the largest port (usually at the umbilicus). The gallbladder bed is irrigated and haemostasis checked. The carbon dioxide is then removed from the abdomen, the fascia closed at the umbilicus and the skin closed.

Laparoscopic cholecystectomy is one of the best examples of minimal access surgery. Minimal access surgery is the same operation through a smaller wound. It encompasses laparoscopy, thoracoscopy, arthroscopy and endoluminal endoscopy. Although these techniques have been around for many years, it is only within the last 20–25 years that laparoscopy has been used for surgical procedures such as laparoscopic cholecystectomy, appendicectomy, fundoplication and hernia repair. More recently, improved instrumentation has seen the acceptance of laparoscopic colectomy and rectal resection, laparoscopic distal pancreatectomy, laparoscopic liver resection and laparoscopic gastrectomy.

The proposed advantages of laparoscopic surgery are attributable to a smaller wound, and hence less postoperative pain, a wound that heals more quickly with less chance of infection, earlier mobilisation and quicker patient recovery.

The disadvantages of laparoscopy include the following: the need for special equipment and extra training, the procedure itself is technically more challenging (hand-eye coordination), the intraoperative complications are harder to deal with (e.g. haemostasis is required as otherwise the blood can obscure the field of vision), and there is loss of tactile feedback. There have also been reports of tumour implantation at port hole sites, but with experience these have reduced and laparoscopic resection is now accepted in the management of malignant disease.

The question as to whether laparoscopic surgery is cost-effective is at present not possible to answer. It involves many factors, including the expertise of the surgeon, the length of the operation, the cost of the hospital stay, better outcomes, and hence remains a debated question and subject of research.

intestine such as usually occurs for a few days after a laparotomy.) It is relatively rare but is frequently asked about in finals.

In the normal anatomical position the gallbladder lies adjacent to the duodenum. A gallstone ileus is caused when a large gallstone (usually >2.5 cm) erodes directly through the wall of the gallbladder into the duodenum. Small gallstones will not cause intestinal obstruction, and they normally enter the duodenum by passing down the cystic duct and then the common bile duct. The erosion of a large gallstone directly into the duodenum is a process which probably occurs over a very long period of time. Surrounding inflammation seals the area such that no local abscess or peritonitis occurs in these cases. Once in the duodenum the stone starts to move down the intestine by peristalsis. The narrowest part of the intestinal tract (after the gastro-oesophageal junction) is about 2 ft proximal to the ileocaecal valve and it is here that the gallstone may impact. The classical X-ray would show the signs of distal small bowel obstruction, air within the biliary tree (because of the fistula between the gallbladder and the duodenum) and the gallstone in the right lower quadrant of the abdomen. Most cases, however, are not diagnosed until surgery. Treatment is removal of the stone through an enterotomy (incision in the small bowel). The gallbladder is usually left alone, as removal can lead to a hole in the duodenum.

CARCINOMA OF THE GALLBLADDER

This is a relatively rare malignancy. Unfortunately, most cases are advanced at the time of presentation. It is associated with long-standing gallstones, polyps of the gallbladder (if a gallbladder polyp is >1 cm in size, then a cholecystectomy should usually be performed) and calcification of the gallbladder (known as a porcelain gallbladder), which is also an indication for cholecystectomy.

Incidental carcinoma of the gallbladder is found in 0.5–1% of laparoscopic cholecystectomies. If suspected preoperatively the patient should be referred to a hepatobiliary surgeon and a radical open cholecystectomy performed. If suspected following removal of the gallbladder at cholecystectomy, a retrieval bag should be used to avoid port site recurrences. In such patients a further radical operation, including resection of the gallbladder bed of the liver, excision of the extrahepatic biliary tree and radical hilar lymphadenectomy should be performed as a second operation if there is no evidence of metastatic disease.

TUMOURS OF THE PANCREAS

Although ductal adenocarcinoma of the pancreas (known as pancreatic cancer) is one of the most lethal of all gastrointestinal tumours, 10–15% of tumours of the pancreas (including those of the periampullary region) are not of the same histological type as ductal carcinoma and have a much better prognosis. This group of tumours includes ampullary carcinoma, islet cell tumours of the pancreas and cystic tumours of the pancreas. A tumour of the pancreas should, therefore, not be assumed to carry a poor prognosis.

Ductal adenocarcinoma of the pancreas is highly malignant and has usually metastasised by the time of diagnosis. Smoking is the only recognised aetiological factor and the disease is uncommon under the age of 40. The disease occurs in the head of the pancreas in 80% of cases and these patients usually present with obstructive jaundice. Pancreatic cancer may also present with severe upper abdominal pain (which may radiate into the back), weight loss, anorexia, malaise or, rarely, thrombophlebitis migrans.

On examination there may be cervical lymphadenopathy, an abdominal mass, hepatomegaly or ascites. The gallbladder may be palpable. Courvoisier's law states that if in the presence of jaundice the gallbladder is palpable, then the cause is unlikely to be gallstones.

Investigations include basic blood tests and specific diagnosis by ultrasound (to detect biliary obstruction), MRCP to exclude stones as the cause of the obstruction and CT to detect and identify the extent of the tumour. EUS gives good views of the pancreas and is used to clarify CT findings and to provide FNA biopsy. ERCP allows therapeutic stent insertion (see section on obstructive jaundice).

Most pancreatic cancers are too advanced for resection at presentation and are treated palliatively by insertion of a biliary stent or bypass surgery. Surgical resection is possible in 15–20% of patients with a ductal carcinoma and in 50–75% of patients with ampullary carcinoma, islet cell tumours or radiate directly through to the back. The patient may also have nausea or vomiting and the condition may rapidly progress to involve the whole abdomen and lead to shock. Usually the abdomen is diffusely tender but soft with normal bowel sounds; however, with significant acute pancreatitis the abdomen can have an appearance similar to peritonitis with the patient preferring to lie still, widespread guarding and rigidity and absent bowel sounds. There is no absolute test for a diagnosis of pancreatitis. The condition should be suspected in cases with such presentation, but sometimes it can be impossible to exclude other causes of the acute abdomen, such as a perforated ulcer, without recourse to laparotomy.

The most useful test is the serum amylase level, but this can be normal in up to 30% of patients. If serum amylase is greater than three times the upper limit of normal, this is usually diagnostic of acute pancreatitis; however, the degree of elevation of the serum amylase does not bear any clear relationship to the severity of the pancreatitis. If a patient is strongly suspected of having acute pancreatitis but the serum amylase is normal, this may be because the earlier onset of symptoms has resulted in the amylase returning to normal. In this case the measurement of serum lipase is useful because this stays elevated longer than the amylase. The measurement of urinary amylase is also useful since this remains elevated for 24–48 h longer than the serum amylase.

In patients still suspected of having acute pancreatitis where diagnosis has not been confirmed, a contrast-enhanced CT scan should be carried out, which will demonstrate acute inflammatory change of the pancreas which may progress to necrosis after a few days. Early assessment of severity in acute pancreatitis is worthwhile because those patients with predicted severe acute pancreatitis should be monitored more closely, considered for prophylactic antibiotics and if the aetiology is gallstones, considered for an urgent ERCP and endoscopic sphincterotomy. Assessment of severity is carried out by a multifactorial scoring system such as the Modified Glasgow Score (Table 5.2). Alternatively, measurement of the C-reactive protein, particularly if carried out as a repeated measurement, can also provide an accurate assessment of severity.

In the initial stages of treatment of acute pancreatitis the aims are resuscitation of the patient with intravenous fluids and oxygen and analgesia. If the patient is vomiting then the patient should be kept nil by

Table 5.2.   Modified Glasgow Score for Acute Pancreatitis

Variable (within 48 h of admission)	Score 1 point if present (a score of 3 or more indicates severe pancreatitis)
Age	Greater than 55 years
pO_2	<8.0 kPa
White blood count	$>15 \times 10^9/l$
Serum calcium (uncorrected)	<2 mmol/l
ALT	>100 IU/l
Serum LDH	>600 IU/l
Blood glucose	>10 mmol/l
Blood urea albumin	>16 mmol/l <32 g/l

Note: This is not the same as the Glasgow Coma Scale used in head injuries.

mouth and a nasogastric tube considered. If the patient is not vomiting then this is not obligatory. Fluid balance charts must be kept and a urinary catheter is necessary to accurately monitor urine output hourly. It is usually necessary to give patients large volumes of fluid intravenously and it is essential that the urine output is maintained above 30 ml/h.

The development of renal failure is associated with a bad prognosis. Respiratory failure in the form of adult respiratory distress syndrome is also associated with a bad prognosis. There is still debate about the precise role of antibiotics in acute pancreatitis. For those patients with predicted severe pancreatitis, most units give prophylactic antibiotics for seven days. Those agents in common usage include meropenem, imipenen, ciprofloxacin and cefuroxime. The use of antibiotics beyond seven days should be in response to positive cultures only. During treatment of acute pancreatitis, gastric acid secretion should be reduced by the administration of a proton pump inhibitor or H2-receptor antagonist. Early assessment of aetiology is also important. Ultrasound is carried out in the first 24 h to look for gallstones and if gallstones are present, the patient will require an elective laparoscopic cholecystectomy to prevent further attacks. If the patient has a biliary cause and also has severe pancreatitis, an urgent endoscopic sphincterotomy should be carried out as this has been shown to reduce mortality in severe acute pancreatitis.

The majority of patients with acute pancreatitis settle down after a few days and make a good recovery. However, in severe acute pancreatitis, patients may die early from multiorgan failure (often respiratory and renal failure). If they get over the acute phase, patients with severe acute pancreatitis may develop infected pancreatic necrosis. This is suspected if the patient has a positive blood culture, if there are changes of low density within the pancreas on CT or if the patient's condition deteriorates with a high white cell count. The presence of infective necrosis can usually be confirmed by CT-guided aspiration. The conventional treatment of infected pancreatic necrosis is open surgery with necrosectomy and postoperative cavity irrigation.

More recently, other techniques have been developed to treat infected necrosis, including percutaneous retroperitoneal necrosectomy, which is performed by a retroperitoneal approach using a modified nephroscope. An alternative technique, which is only suitable for walled-off collections behind the stomach, is transgastric endoscopic necrosectomy, which is carried out under endoscopic ultrasound guidance. Infected necrosis is the most common cause of late death in acute pancreatitis. If the necrosis does not become infected, other complications may occur, such as pseudocyst formation. A pseudocyst is a collection of fluid in the lesser peritoneal sac. If a pseudocyst is persistent, drainage may be necessary and this can usually be carried out endoscopically. Occasionally, laparoscopic or open cyst-gastrostomy may be necessary.

Nutrition is a very important aspect of the management of acute pancreatitis. The majority of patients can be fed enterally from early on in the illness and enteral nutrition is associated with a reduction in complications in acute pancreatitis. Feeding is usually achieved by placement of a nasojejunal feeding tube.

OBSTRUCTIVE JAUNDICE

Jaundice can be classified in three ways. The most common is to divide it into prehepatic (such as is caused by haemolytic anaemia), hepatic (caused by hepatitis) and posthepatic jaundice (which is also called obstructive jaundice). Prehepatic and hepatic causes of jaundice are usually dealt with as medical conditions not requiring surgery and will not be referred to further in this chapter.

An additional type of obstructive jaundice should, however, be mentioned, namely drug-induced cholestatic jaundice, which is produced by drugs such as chlorpromazine. Clinically and biochemically this can be impossible to differentiate from true obstructive jaundice without further tests, and it is important that all cases of jaundice have a careful drug history taken.

The classical symptoms of obstructive jaundice are, first of all, the yellow appearance of the skin and mucous membranes. Quite often patients will have had this pointed out to them by a friend or relative rather than noticing it themselves. In addition they may have noticed a change in their urine and stools, with the urine becoming darker and the stools becoming paler. The urine becomes darker because conjugated bilirubin appears in it and the stool becomes paler because no bilirubin is entering the bowel. In addition the patients may complain of itching, which is caused by the deposition of bile salts in the skin (not bilirubin!). Pain is a variable feature in posthepatic obstructive jaundice. It is more common when jaundice is caused by gallstones. But it may still be a feature even with obstruction due to carcinoma at the head of the pancreas. These two entities, gallstones and carcinoma of the pancreas, are the main areas to be discussed when answering questions about obstructive jaundice in surgical finals, as they each constitute about one third of the causes of obstructive jaundice (the other third of the causes are cholangiocarcinoma, chronic pancreatitis and enlarged lymph nodes in the porta hepatis).

Clinical Assessment

Clinical assessment of obstructive jaundice consists, first of all, of taking a full history. The importance in noting any drug therapy has been mentioned above. The duration of symptoms, associated weight loss (which can be particularly marked in obstructive jaundice, due to difficulty in fat and vitamin absorption), as well as the specific features of obstructive jaundice (itching, pale stools, dark urine), should be noted. Physical examination will reveal jaundice itself. Jaundice is usually best seen by examining the sclerae of the eyes. Bilirubin levels above 50 μmol/l are usually clinically detectable (the normal range is up to 17 μmol/l). Other features to look for on physical examination include the stigmata of chronic liver disease (spider naevi, liver palms, Dupuytren's contracture, liver flap, gynaecomastia, testicular atrophy, etc.).

Examination of the abdomen should look for enlargement or tenderness of the liver and the presence of ascites. If the gallbladder is palpable, then Courvoisier's law should be considered. This law states that if in the presence of jaundice the gallbladder is palpable, then the cause of jaundice is unlikely to be gallstones. The reason for this law is that when gallstones have been present for a significant period of time, chronic cholecystitis results in a thickening fibrosis of the gallbladder wall, making it unable to distend even when obstruction occurs. An exception is when there is dual pathology. A distended gallbladder will be felt underneath the right costal margin as a smooth, convex, perhaps slightly tender mass which moves down with the liver with inspiration.

Basic investigations in patients with jaundice will include full blood count, U&E, liver function tests and a chest X-ray. The liver function tests will confirm the obstructive nature of the jaundice. Bilirubin will be raised, but the specific liver enzyme that will be raised predominantly is alkaline phosphatase rather than the transaminases. In addition, all jaundice patients should have their baseline clotting status checked.

The next most important test is the ultrasound scan, which is a quick and cheap way of demonstrating whether there is extrahepatic biliary obstruction, whether gallstones are present and perhaps whether there is a tumour in the pancreas. Ultrasound is very good at determining dilatation of the biliary tree and common bile duct (the normal maximum upper limit for the width of the common bile duct is 7 mm). A diameter of up to 1.1 cm may be normal if there was previous obstruction which has now resolved. A width of the common bile duct greater than 1.1 cm is likely to be abnormal. Ultrasound is also very good at looking at the gallbladder and for the presence of gallstones. Unfortunately the lower end of the common bile duct and the head of the pancreas are often poorly seen on ultrasound, due to overlying bowel gas. This is a particular problem in overweight patients. If further imaging is felt to be needed, then the type of imaging will depend on the findings at ultrasound. The options for further treatment are probably best illustrated by describing certain clinical examples.

*Example 1: Obstructive Jaundice with a Stone in the Bile Duct on
Ultrasound*

In this situation, ultrasound has clearly shown a stone in the bile duct
and this is likely to be the cause of the obstruction. There are two ways
of dealing with this scenario. One option is laparoscopic cholecystectomy and laparoscopic common bile duct exploration, a combination of
procedures that is favoured by advanced laparoscopic surgeons. An
alternative would be ERCP and stone extraction followed by laparoscopic cholecystectomy. ERCP should only be done if therapy is to be
carried out since complications may be serious (see subsection on
ERCP). In the case of a stone, an endoscopic sphincterotomy is performed and the stone removed using a basket or balloon. Open surgery
for common bile duct stones is now performed rarely but may
occasionally be necessary if the stones cannot be removed laparoscopically or endoscopically. In this case, the common bile duct is
opened between stay sutures, the stones removed and either a T-tube
placed in the common bile duct or the duct closed primarily. A T-tube
is inserted, a T-tube cholangiogram is carried out ten days after the
operation and if the duct is clear the T-tube can then be removed 14
days after surgery.

*Example 2: Obstructive Jaundice, Ultrasound Showing a Dilated
Common Bile Duct Down to the Head of the Pancreas*

In this situation, where obstructive jaundice is present but no gallstones
have been seen, the patient is suspected of harbouring a tumour of the
head of the pancreas or ampulla of Vater. The next test should be a contrast-enhanced CT scan with fine cuts through the upper abdomen to look
closely at the liver, biliary tract and pancreas. If a mass is present then features of unresectability (liver metastases, lymph node metastases or
involvement of the portal vein or superior mesenteric vein or artery)
should be sought. If none of these features of unresectability are present,
the patient should proceed to an endoscopic ultrasound (see subsection on
EUS). If EUS suggests that the patient has an operable tumour, then the
patient should ideally undergo surgery, if fit, before the bilirubin climbs

Infection

Patients with obstructive jaundice appear to have a greater incidence of infection problems, including wound complications. This may be partly due to their poor protein status and there is a non-specific effect of malignancy on the immune system. The patient should be appropriately covered with broad-spectrum antibiotics, preferably those which appear in the bile.

Cholangitis

Cholangitis is one of the most feared complications in obstructive jaundice. It is the cause of Charcot's triad, which consists of rigors or fever, abdominal pain and jaundice. It is caused by infection within an obstructed biliary tree. It should be regarded as an emergency, as left untreated it can result in severe shock, renal failure and death.

LIVER TUMOURS

The majority of liver tumours are secondary tumours metastasised from elsewhere, particularly from primary tumours of the gastrointestinal tract. In a patient presenting with a mass in the liver, it is therefore important to take a careful history of previous malignancy, underlying liver disease, previous surgery that may have been for cancer and to examine the patient thoroughly for the presence of malignancy and evidence of parenchymal liver disease such as cirrhosis.

Routine blood tests are important, especially LFTs, tumour markers and, if necessary, serological and immunological markers of liver disease. An ultrasound is the first imaging test to be done. This will show whether the lesion is solid or cystic. A small cyst can usually be ignored or followed up. A larger cyst may need further investigation. Hydatid, a parasitic cystic disease caused by *Echinococcus*, can be excluded by a laboratory (ELISA) test. Larger cysts may also be biliary cystadenomas which sometimes need excision. If the ultrasound shows a solid lesion, this implies a tumour and further detailed investigation is necessary. A full CT of the chest, abdomen and pelvis should be carried out. A primary gastrointestinal tumour may be seen but a colonoscopy and gastroscopy may be required. A solitary liver lesion may be a primary liver tumour such as hepatocellular carcinoma or hepatic adenoma (rare and associated with the oral contraceptive pill). If associated with cirrhosis the prognosis will usually depend on the underlying liver disease. If the uninvolved liver is normal, resection should be considered.

The presence of multiple solid liver lesions usually implies disseminated malignancy. It is unusual for multiple liver metastases to be suitable for surgical resection but this may be appropriate in colorectal cancer and in other cancers which are slow growing, such as neuroendocrine tumours. Solitary solid lesions are not so common but are often suitable for resection. A primary tumour should be sought avidly by CT and endoscopy. Then tumours suitable for resection can be carefully imaged by MRI, which is a good technique for detailed liver imaging. Secondary colorectal tumours identified after resection of the primary tumour can be imaged and then resected, provided there is no unresectable disease elsewhere in the body. The use of positron emission tomography (PET) scans is advisable to exclude tumours elsewhere. If identified at the same time as the primary tumour, it is usually appropriate to resect the primary tumour first and to repeat the CT to ensure the liver disease is resectable before undertaking a separate liver resection. Chemotherapy has a definite role to play and other treatments such as radiofrequency ablation may be appropriate.

6

DISORDERS OF THE OESOPHAGUS, STOMACH AND DUODENUM

Sarah Robinson and S Michael Griffin

Disorders of the oesophagus, stomach and duodenum are dealt with by medical and surgical gastroenterologists. It is the aspects of these disorders relating to surgery which are discussed in this chapter. Most upper gastrointestinal (GI) conditions give rise to symptoms rather than signs, and upper GI endoscopy is the mainstay of diagnosis.

DYSPHAGIA

Dysphagia is defined as difficulty in swallowing, whilst pain on swallowing is known as odynophagia. Most disorders of the oesophagus that are of relevance to surgical finals have dysphagia as a presenting symptom. Table 6.1 lists the most common causes and subdivides them into intraluminal, intra- and extramural and systemic causes.

The mainstays of investigation of dysphagia include endoscopy, barium swallow and manometric assessment.

- *Endoscopy*. Investigation of choice. Allows visual assessment, biopsy and histological review with the option for therapeutic intervention.
- *Barium swallow*. Minimally invasive. Allows assessment of motility disorders in the absence of endoscopic findings.
- *Manometry*. Adjunct to endoscopy and barium swallow. Provides detailed assessment of the lower oesophageal sphincter and oesophageal peristalsis. This is of particular importance in achalasia.

Table 6.1.   Causes of Dysphagia

Intraluminal (inside the lumen)
    Foreign body bolus obstruction (children and psychiatric patients)
    Polypoid tumours
    Oesophageal inflammation (oesophagitis)
    Oesophageal infection (candidiasis, herpes simplex)
Extraluminal (outside the lumen)
Intramural (in the wall)
    Benign strictures (gastro-oesophageal reflux, ingestion of caustic substances)
    Malignant strictures
    Achalasia
    Oesophageal web (Plummer–Vinson syndrome: middle-aged females with iron
        deficiency anaemia. The web consists of desquamated epithelium)
    Nutcracker oesophagus (characterised by high-pressure contractions with normal
        peristalsis on manometry)
    Diffuse oesophageal spasm
    Scleroderma
    Presbyoesophagus (dysmotility associated with old age)
Extramural (outside the wall, pressing in)
    Pharyngeal pouch
    Rolling hiatus hernia
    Malignancy (lung and mediastinal)
    Retrosternal goitre
    Vascular structures: thoracic aortic aneurysms, congenitally abnormal vessels
        (dysphagia lusoria)
Systemic causes
    Myasthenia gravis
    Multiple sclerosis
    Parkinson's disease
    Pseudobulbar palsy
    Psychological

OESOPHAGEAL CANCER

The incidence of oesophageal cancer is increasing faster than any other solid organ malignancy in the Western world. It is now the eighth commonest malignancy in the UK. The oesophagus is normally lined by squamous epithelium but gastric-type mucosa, termed Barrett's oesophagus, may develop at the lower end. In recent years the relative incidence of squamous and adenocarcinoma have changed dramatically. Although previously squamous predominated, adenocarcinomas now account for 65% of all oesophageal carcinomas in the UK. Most patients are middle-aged or elderly, with a male to female ratio of 3:1.

Barrett's oesophagus is a condition in which the normal squamous epithelium in the distal oesophagus is replaced with glandular epithelium (columnar epithelium). It is usually secondary to gastro-oesophageal reflux and is associated with an increased risk of developing oesophageal adeno-carcinoma. Consequently, many units adopt an endoscopic surveillance programme to detect malignant changes at an early stage. Other risk factors include obesity, high dietary fat intake, smoking, alcohol and male Caucasian origin. The principal risk factors for squamous carcinoma are alcohol intake and tobacco use. The incidence is increased in Northern China, Iran and South Africa in comparison to Western countries. In addition, diets rich in nitrosamines and deficient in vitamins A and C and trace elements, achala-sia, caustic strictures, hereditary tylosis (an autosomal dominant genetic disorder characterised by hyperkeratosis of the soles and palms and oral leukoplakia) and coexisting aerodigestive tract cancers are all implicated.

Most oesophageal cancers present with dysphagia, by which time spread has often occurred through the wall of the oesophagus and to lymph nodes. Without treatment the average survival from diagnosis is nine months. Dysphagia is usually progressive: initially to solids (espe-cially bread) and then liquids. Patients will often alter their dietary habits to increase their intake of liquids and soft foods in the earlier stages. This exacerbates the weight loss normally associated with malignancy. Significant weight loss is therefore common at presentation. Oesophageal obstruction may lead to overflow of the oesophageal contents, in turn pre-disposing to aspiration pneumonia. This risk is greatest at night when the patient is supine. Physical examination may reveal lymphadenopathy or hepatomegaly and ascites, but often there will be no abnormalities to detect other than obvious weight loss.

The mainstay of investigation is upper GI endoscopy. This allows biopsy or cytological examination of any lesions to confirm the diagnosis. In addition, dilatations, under X-ray control, can be performed to ease the symptoms of dysphagia. The patient will then undergo a more thorough staging process, including computed tomography (CT) scanning and endoscopic ultrasound (a special ultrasound probe attached to the endoscope) to assess invasion of adjacent structures and help predict resectability. Patient fitness is determined and further tests, including bone scanning, magnetic resonance imaging (MRI) and positron emission tomography (PET) scanning, may also need to be performed. This will allow the stage of the tumour to be determined, which will dictate the treatment options available. Staging uses the internationally recognised TNM method (i.e. tumour, node, metastases — see p. 141).

The aim of treatment in carcinoma of the oesophagus is cure where possible and palliation where not. Surgery, where feasible, offers the greatest opportunity for cure. However, as a consequence of the advanced stage of the disease at presentation and the patient's coexisting disease (comorbidity), only one third of patients have a technically resectable tumour at presentation. There is no role for palliative surgery in patients with proven distant metastases. There are several surgical approaches to resection of the oesophagus (oesophagectomy). The principle is to resect all macroscopic tumour and mobilise the stomach so that it can be brought up into the chest or neck for anastomosis to the remaining oesophagus. To achieve this, abdominal, chest (thoracotomy) and neck incisions may be required. Neoadjuvant chemotherapy is now the standard of care for those patients with advanced but potentially curable cancer, following the publication of the OEO2 and MAGIC chemotherapy trials. A full restaging is performed postchemotherapy to assess response prior to undertaking surgical resection. At least two thirds of all staged patients will be inoperable, requiring palliative treatment. Repeated dilatations, oesophageal stenting, tumour ablation with laser or argon beam, chemotherapy and radiotherapy can be used to provide relief of dysphagia. Radiotherapy may be performed externally or within the lumen of the oesophagus (brachytherapy).

The prognosis for oesophageal cancer is poor. Surgically treated patients have stage-dependent survival. Palliatively treated patients have a median survival of four months. Overall five-year survival is 10–15%.

GASTRIC CANCER

Gastric cancer is one of the most common cancers in the world. This is due to a high prevalence in East Asia and South America. The incidence in Western populations has actually decreased over recent decades. In the UK it is currently the sixth commonest cancer. In addition, the commonest site of gastric cancer has altered from distal to proximal (cardia) over the previous three decades. The majority of gastric cancers are adenocarcinomas. Three percent are lymphomas and less commonly gastrointestinal stromal tumours and neuroendocrine tumours.

Risk factors for developing gastric cancer include *Helicobacter pylori* colonisation, blood group A, smoking and diet. A high dietary intake of nitrate- and salt-containing foods, associated with pickling methods, is linked to gastric cancer, whereas increased vitamin C consumption is thought to be protective. There is an increased risk associated with pernicious anaemia and previous gastric surgery. A few cases of familial gastric cancer have been identified which are associated with abnormalities of E-cadherin (a cellular adhesion molecule) expression.

Gastric cancer is classified in several ways. Early or late describes the depth of invasion of the tumour. Early gastric cancer (EGC) is confined to the mucosa or submucosa. In the late form the muscularis propria is breached. The incidence of EGC is 10% in the West and 40% in Japan. Histologically, gastric cancer is described as intestinal or diffuse, the latter having a worse prognosis. Linitis plastica (leather bottle stomach) is the description applied to diffuse gastric cancer affecting the entire stomach wall. Endoscopically this is recognisable as a non-distending stomach. Transcoelomic spread, throughout the peritoneal cavity, can occur with a predilection for the ovaries (Krukenberg tumour).

In the West, presentation is typically late and most often includes a history of weight loss and anorexia, epigastric pain, nausea and vomiting. Less commonly, patients may present with upper gastrointestinal bleeding or gastric perforation. Abdominal examination may reveal an epigastric mass, a succussion splash (splashing of residual gastric fluid, caused by an obstructing antral cancer), ascites or hepatomegaly. A left supraclavicular lymph node may be palpable (Virchow's node); when present this is known as Troisier's sign. Another association is with acanthosis nigricans (pigmented warty axillary skin). Pelvic deposits may be felt on rectal examination. These findings all indicate very advanced disease.

Diagnosis is made endoscopically, at which time confirmatory biopsies may be taken. Further staging takes the form of thoracic and abdominal CT, endoscopic ultrasound and laparoscopy, with some patients undergoing bone scans. PET scanning is rarely useful in gastric cancer.

Various treatment options exist depending on the stage of the tumour and the fitness of the patient. The options include the following:

- *Surgery*. This can be curative or palliative. As with oesophageal cancer, surgery, where feasible, offers the greatest opportunity for cure. However, unlike oesophageal cancer, surgery has a palliative role in the treatment of gastric cancer. Obstructing and bleeding tumours may be treated with bypass procedures or palliative resections in an otherwise fit individual. With curative surgery, operation type is dictated by the position of the tumour. In most proximal tumours a total gastrectomy is undertaken but in more distal cases a subtotal gastrectomy is possible. A Roux-en-Y anastomosis is usually performed to prevent bile reflux. Early gastric cancers may be treated with endoscopic resection.
- *Chemotherapy*. The role of chemotherapy is predominantly palliative but research into neoadjuvant and intraperitoneal chemotherapy is ongoing.
- *Endoscopic and medical palliation*. Endoscopically placed pyloric stents (passage of a plastic tube through the tumour to allow drainage of the stomach) may be used to relieve obstructive symptoms. Proton pump inhibitors can reduce bleeding from ulcerating gastric tumours. Argon plasma coagulation (APC), a method of electrocoagulation using high-frequency electrical energy to achieve tissue destruction and haemostasis, is useful in the palliative treatment of polypoid gastric tumours.
- *Radiotherapy*. This is of no value.

Overall, five-year survival of patients with gastric cancer in the UK is still in the region of 10%. Gastric cancer is often used as a classic model for the way in which tumours spread, namely:

- Spread within the wall of the organ, leading to the so-called linitis plastica
- Local spread to adjacent structures, such as the pancreas
- Lymphatic spread to local lymph nodes and further afield
- Transcoelomic spread, where the tumour seeds across the peritoneal cavity
- Blood-borne spread such as occurs with lung metastases

GASTROINTESTINAL STROMAL TUMOURS (GISTs)

Mesenchymal tumours of the GI tract originate within the bowel wall. They are divided into three groups with varying differentiation of neural and smooth muscle expression by immunohistochemistry.

- Leiomyomas and leiomyosarcomas express markers of smooth muscle differentiation.
- Neurofibromas are positive for S100, indicating a neural origin.
- GISTs are positive for CD34 and CD117 (c-Kit protein) and originate from the interstitial cells of Cajal: the pacemaker cells of the GI tract. They comprise the largest group.

GISTs occur most commonly within the stomach (60–70%) and are rare within the oesophagus (2–3%) where leiomyomas predominate. They usually occur over the age of 40 with an equal male to female ratio. Three quarters are benign with indicators of malignancy including tumour size >10 cm, location (extragastric position), mitotic index >5/10 high-power fields and evidence of cystic degeneration on endoscopic ultrasound.

Many are found incidentally but may present as abdominal pain, GI bleeding or with obstructive symptoms. Endoscopically they appear as well-demarcated spherical masses often with a central punctum. Superficial surface erosion may occur. Treatment is surgical resection based on clinical indications. These include size and physiological effects such as obstruction and clinically significant bleeding. Imatinib and more recently sumatinib, Kit-selective tyrosine kinase inhibitors, have demonstrated success in the treatment of metastatic c-Kit-positive GISTs.

PHARYNGEAL POUCH

A pharyngeal pouch (also known as Zenker's diverticulum) is an out-pouching of the pharynx, usually between the upper border of the cricopharyngeus muscle and the lower border of the inferior constrictor muscle of the pharynx. This corresponds with a weak area called Killian's dehiscence.

Pharyngeal pouches are thought to be pulsion diverticulae, caused by peristaltic activity pumping against resistance resulting from uncoordinated muscle spasms. Although the deficit occurs posteriorly, any associated swelling usually bulges to the left side of the neck and may produce a palpable lump on examination. Food debris may collect within the diverticulum, which can in turn expand, pressing on the adjacent oesophagus, causing dysphagia. Patients may also complain of regurgitation of food from the diverticulum, gurgling sounds or bad breath (halitosis) due to the presence of decaying food in the diverticulum. Sometimes a patient will learn to empty the pouch by using external pressure on the neck. A further complication of oesophageal pouches is perforation at endoscopy should the scope enter the diverticulum rather than the oesophagus. Surgical treatment options include simple excision of the pouch by an open surgical approach. Endoscopic stapling of the bridge between the pouch and the oesophagus, opening up the pouch and allowing it to drain more freely, is increasingly considered the treatment of choice.

PERFORATION OF THE OESOPHAGUS

Oesophageal perforation may be caused by trauma at endoscopy or by ingestion of a sharp foreign body, such as a fish bone. Spontaneous rupture of the oesophagus (Boerhaave's syndrome) occurs with forceful or prolonged vomiting. Ingestion of corrosive agents (acids/alkalis) and penetrating chest injuries are less common causes. Perforation will result in mediastinitis (infection and inflammation of the mediastinum as a result of food/fluid/micro-organisms entering the mediastinum). Prompt diagnosis is essential, taking the form of plain chest X-ray, contrast swallow, endoscopy and CT, to evaluate the extent and position of the perforation. Iatrogenic perforations can usually be managed conservatively, due to minimal levels of contamination, with a nasogastric tube for gastric decompression, a nasojejunal tube for nutrition purposes, proton pump inhibitors and antibiotics, including antifungals. Most other perforations require resuscitation of the patient who is usually very unwell as diagnosis is often delayed. In addition to the above treatment, surgery to debride the mediastinum and placement of a T-tube within the oesophagus, to provide drainage and the formation of a controlled oesophagocutaneous fistula, is the mainstay of treatment. The oesophagus should rarely be repaired in the first instance in the presence of pleural soiling.

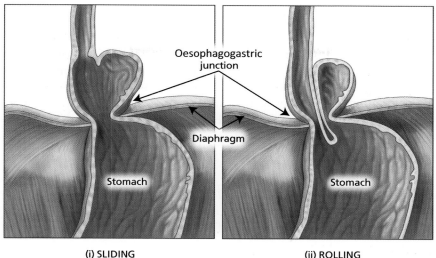

(i) SLIDING   (ii) ROLLING

Figure 6.1.   The two main types of hiatus hernia.

REFLUX DISEASE AND HIATUS HERNIA

The oesophagus passes into the abdomen from the thorax through the oesophageal hiatus of the diaphragm. Normally about 2–4 cm of the oesophagus lies within the abdomen. Hiatus hernias may either be sliding (85%), rolling (10%) or mixed (5%) (Figure 6.1). With a sliding hiatus hernia the oesophagogastric junction moves up into the thorax. The oesophagogastric junction is in the normal position with a rolling hiatus hernia which is caused by the stomach rolling up beside the oesophagus.

Hiatus hernia commonly presents with retrosternal burning pains which may be worse on bending, stooping or at night on lying flat. Such symptoms are often called heartburn by patients and are due to the reflux of gastric contents (predominantly acid) into the oesophagus. This is termed gastro-oesophageal reflux disease (GORD). Regurgitation of acid fluid into the mouth may occur (water brash). Patients will normally report increased pain after meals (postprandially) and will usually have noticed some relief with proprietary over-the-counter antacids. Severe reflux oesophagitis may lead to ulceration and bleeding or, if long-standing, benign stricture formation.

Treatment of hiatus hernia involves measures such as losing weight, stopping smoking, eating smaller meals earlier in the evening and raising the head of the bed. Antacids, H2-receptor antagonists, proton pump inhibitors and drugs which mechanically prevent reflux by forming a protective layer on top of the contents of the stomach, such as some of the alginate preparations, may be helpful. Where medical therapy has failed or where the patient is unhappy with the prospect of permanent medication, surgery may be indicated. Many operations have been described but the commonest is the floppy Nissen fundoplication. This involves mobilising the fundus of the stomach and wrapping it around the lower end of the oesophagus, providing a high-pressure area to prevent reflux. This operation is increasingly performed laparoscopically.

Prior to the surgical treatment of reflux it is important to perform pH and manometry studies. This will exclude a diagnosis of achalasia or dysmotility prior to performing a wrap. In addition, 24-hour ambulatory oesophageal pH assessment confirms the diagnosis of GORD.

ACHALASIA OF THE OESOPHAGUS

This is due to failure of relaxation of the smooth muscle at the lower end of the oesophagus secondary to an abnormality of its nerve supply. It usually presents in middle age and the precise cause is unknown. It has some similarities to the tropical disease trypanosomiasis (Chagas disease), in which the nerve supply to the oesophageal muscle is also deficient. It usually presents with intermittent dysphagia with gradual progression. The patient may complain of fluid regurgitation, which tends to be worse at night, and is associated with pneumonia due to aspiration. Diagnosis is made on barium swallow with the typical features of a dilated oesophagus above a smooth tapering with a "bird's beak" appearance. Oesophageal manometry provides manometric confirmation of a non-relaxing sphincter. Achalasia is treated either by endoscopic dilatation of the lower oesophageal sphincter under X-ray control or by an operation termed a Heller's procedure in conjunction with an antireflux procedure. The former is a cardiomyotomy, i.e. an operation which involves dividing the muscle layer at the lower end of the oesophagus and entrance of the stomach (cardia) down as far as the mucosa. The mucosa is left intact. It is similar in principle to the Ramstedt's operation for infantile hyper-trophic pyloric stenosis. Squamous carcinoma of the oesophagus develops in 3–5% of patients with achalasia.

PEPTIC ULCERATION

Peptic ulceration is defined as ulcer formation associated with acid and can occur at several sites, namely the duodenum (commonest), stomach, oesophagus, jejunum (in Zollinger–Ellison syndrome), Meckel's divertic-ulum (if it contains ectopic gastric mucosa) and sometimes at the site of a previous gastroenterostomy. Obviously duodenal and stomach ulcers form the vast majority of those cases seen clinically. However, in an essay answer it is important to be able to discuss these other areas if only in broad outline. Peptic ulcer disease, at any site, can present as the following:

- Pain (dyspepsia/indigestion)
- Bleeding (acute or chronic)
- Penetration into adjacent structures (into the pancreas for a posterior duodenal ulcer, gastrocolic fistula)
- Perforation (usually an anterior duodenal or gastric ulcer)
- Obstruction (i.e. severe scarring of the pylorus from chronic ulcera-tion or acute obstruction of the pylorus from acute ulceration with oedema)

H. pylori gastric colonisation is the most important aetiological factor implicated in peptic ulcer disease. Of patients infected with *H. pylori*, 10% will progress to ulcer development. The mechanism of injury is thought to be twofold. A combination of the effects of toxins released by the bacteria and the body's inflammatory response to this leads to direct injury of the protective gastric mucosal barrier. Second, the associated gastritis and pat-terns of gastric recolonisation by *H. pylori* is associated with increased gastrin-induced acid production. This effect is exacerbated by reduced pro-duction of the inhibiting peptide, somatostatin, due to a diminished D-cell mass associated with antral gastritis. More recently, different substrains of *H. pylori* have been identified. These are associated with differing effects on the gastric mucosa: gastritis, gastritis and ulceration or complicated ulcer disease. Host factors play a role. Lewis antibodies on the surface of gastric epithelial cells preferentially bind *H. pylori*. Lewis antibody involvement in the determination of the O blood group may explain a long-recognised association between peptic ulcer disease and this blood type. Host inflammatory response will dictate the degree of mucosal damage elicited by *H. pylori*.

Non-steroidal anti-inflammatory drug (NSAID) use is the second most common factor implicated in ulcer development. Smoking, increased acid secretion, coffee consumption and comorbidity such as liver and renal failure and hyperparathyroidism have all been implicated in the severity of the disease.

Duodenal ulceration occurs most frequently in men and peaks in the 45–55 age group. Gastric ulceration tends to present later with a peak at 55–65 years of age. Ninety-five percent of duodenal ulcers occur in the first part of the duodenum: within 2 cm of the pylorus. Patients often describe pain as being eased by food (unlike gastric ulcers, where it is often worsened by food). The pain is usually worse at night and may radiate through to the back.

Patients with dyspepsia should undergo endoscopic assessment to confirm the presence of an ulcer and to test for the presence of *H. pylori*. Biopsy of all gastric ulcers is essential to avoid missing early gastric cancers. Repeat endoscopy following treatment is advisable to assess healing. Those colonised with *H. pylori* should undergo eradication therapy (proton pump inhibitor and antibiotic regime). NSAIDs and aspirin should be stopped and alternatives prescribed. Cessation of smoking should be encouraged. With this regime the majority of duodenal ulcers can be medically managed and relatively few progress to surgery.

GASTRIC AND DUODENAL ULCER SURGERY

Since the advent of medical management of peptic ulcer disease with H2-receptor antagonists and more recently proton pump inhibitors, and with the eradication of *H. pylori*, surgical treatment is predominantly of historical interest.

You may encounter patients who have undergone surgical treatment of peptic ulcer disease and are now experiencing the long-term complications.

In the surgical examination, in-depth knowledge of gastric physiology will not be required. However, the following principles are important. First, without acid there can be no ulcer formation and, in broad terms, whether or not an ulcer develops is the result of the balance between acid secretion and the mucosal protective factors which are reduced by drugs such as NSAIDs. Remember that the stomach starts at the oesophagogastric junction (cardia). The fundus, body and antrum lead, via the pylorus, into the duodenum. The fundus and body contain cells that produce the acid, pepsinogen and intrinsic factor, whereas the major site of gastrin formation is in the antrum. Most peptic ulceration is found within the first part of the duodenum but may spread further down into the small bowel in Zollinger–Ellison syndrome (see p. 122).

Gastric acid secretion is stimulated by either gastrin or vagal nerve stimulation. There are two vagus nerves supplying the stomach, i.e. the right and the left vagus, which actually sit in a posterior and an anterior position close to the oesophagus as it enters the abdomen. Smaller divisions of the vagus nerves, called the nerves of Latarjet, supply the pyloric region and are responsible for relaxation of the pylorus to allow emptying of the stomach. Other branches of these nerves supply the acid-secreting areas of the stomach. This explains why a truncal vagotomy (division of the vagus nerves as they enter the abdomen) results in reduced acid secretion but a stomach which fails to empty adequately. A truncal vagotomy operation, therefore, needs to be combined with a further procedure to enable emptying of the stomach, such as a pyloroplasty (Figure 6.2) or a gastroenterostomy (Figure 6.3).

Previously performed operations include the following:

- *Truncal or selective vagotomy.* The former requires a drainage procedure, as explained.
- *Antrectomy with vagotomy.* In this procedure the distal half of the stomach is removed (i.e. a partial gastrectomy) in combination with a vagotomy (Figure 6.4). The stomach can then be reanastomosed either directly to the duodenum (Billroth I procedure) or the duodenal stump can be closed over and a small bowel loop brought up for anastomosis onto the stomach (Billroth II procedure, also known as a Polya gastrectomy).

- *Subtotal gastrectomy with Roux-en-Y to restore intestinal continuity.* This involves transecting the small bowel, moving the distal portion proximally to anastomose to the remaining stomach. The end of the proximal section of the small bowel is then reattached approximately 50 cm down this anastomosed segment. Consequently, bile and pancreatic juices enter the small bowel 50 cm downstream from the anastomosis; this is both more physiological and reduces bile reflux.

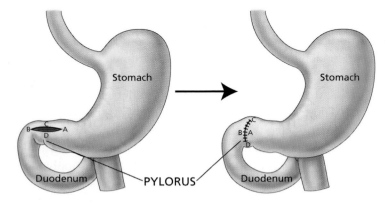

Figure 6.2. Pyloroplasty. A longditudinal incision (A–B) is made through the pylorus and then closed transversely (C–D) to widen it.

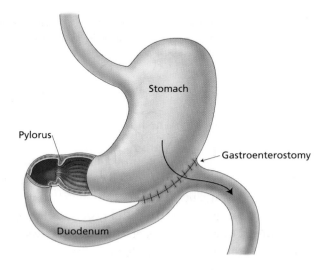

Figure 6.3. Gastroenterostomy.

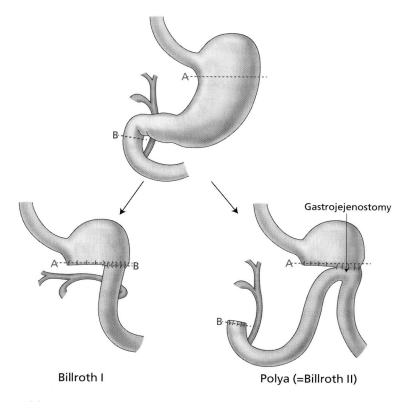

Figure 6.4. Gastrectomies. The distal part of the stomach (between A–A and B–B) is removed and the two main techniques for joining it up again are shown.

The latter operation is still occasionally performed for refractory ulcer disease or in the case of Zollinger–Ellison syndrome (see p. 122).

COMPLICATIONS OF PEPTIC ULCER SURGERY

Although peptic ulcer surgery is nowadays rarely performed, the complications are specific and sometimes discussed in final exams. There are numerous ways of classifying these, an example of which is given below. Remember that complications can be general, applying to any operation, or specific to a particular operation. The following shows in detail only the specific complications related to peptic ulcer operations.

misleadingly normal if the patient has not undergone fluid resuscitation prior to testing. A urinary catheter should be sited to monitor urine output (>30 ml/h). Correction of coagulopathies and prescription of intravenous proton pump inhibitors to decrease the gastric pH should be undertaken. Depending upon the severity of the bleeding, further invasive monitoring (e.g. central venous catheterisation) may be necessary: such patients should be managed in a high dependency unit.

The group with the highest mortality risk from upper gastrointestinal bleeding are those patients who rebleed as inpatients. Risk factors for this include patient age greater than 80 years, shock at presentation, haemoglobin less than 8 g/dl, endoscopic stigmas of recent bleeding and patient comorbidity. Scoring systems have been devised to identify those most at risk (the Rockall score and more recently the Blatchford score).

Endoscopy is now the mainstay of treatment. This is performed to establish a diagnosis and to allow endoscopic intervention to stop the bleeding. This may take the form of injection therapy (adrenaline 1:10,000) which is the most established and frequently used method. Recent developments have included the use of thermal coagulation, laser ablation, fibrin glue application or the use of endoclips.

The indications for urgent surgical intervention include failure to stop the bleeding endoscopically and rebleeding during the current hospital admission. Surgery usually consists of opening the stomach or duodenum and underrunning the bleeding vessel. Postoperatively, patients should undergo *H. pylori* eradication therapy and be commenced on long-term acid suppression medication. All NSAID medication should be stopped.

The initial treatment of bleeding oesophageal varices, following resuscitation and correction of coagulopathies, is endoscopic band ligation or injection sclerotherapy. If this fails to control the bleeding, a Sengstaken tube should be inserted. This comprises two balloons: the gastric to anchor the tube and the oesophageal to tamponade the bleeding sites. The patient will require transfer to a specialist centre for further treatment.

PERFORATED PEPTIC ULCER

The commonest site of peptic ulcer perforation is the duodenum. The usual site for perforation is anteriorly within the first part of the duodenum (posterior perforation is more likely to either penetrate into the pancreas or erode the gastroduodenal artery, causing haemorrhage). Surprisingly, many patients presenting with a perforated peptic ulcer have had little in the way of pre-existing symptoms of indigestion. Presentation is usually sudden in onset with severe epigastric pain and some vomiting. On examination the patient tends to lie very still, avoiding abdominal movement. Tenderness is initially in the epigastrium but will spread throughout the abdomen if the leak is not contained. The abdomen may be rigid with rebound, percussion tenderness and absent bowel sounds. The key investigation is an erect chest X-ray (not an abdominal X-ray). In 70% of cases this will demonstrate gas under the diaphragm.

Treatment involves adequate resuscitation of the patient prior to proceeding to theatre for laparotomy. With a simple duodenal perforation, peritoneal washout and simple closure of the deficit, with a re-enforcing omental patch, is the treatment of choice. In the case of gastric ulcer perforation it is advisable to excise the ulcer with a small ellipse of stomach and then repair the defect. The specimen should then be sent for histological assessment to exclude malignancy: up to one third of perforated gastric ulcers are malignant. Ninety percent of peptic perforations are associated with *H. pylori* and as such eradication therapy with long-term acid suppression treatment is recommended.

HYPERTROPHIC PYLORIC STENOSIS

This condition affects 1–3 in 1000 live births. The male to female ratio is 4:1 with a preponderance of the first-born male. There is an increased prevalence in Caucasian populations and is three times more likely if the child has a positive maternal history. The most common presentation is of vomiting 3–10 weeks postdelivery, which may become projectile in nature. This will be associated with hypokalaemic, hypochloraemic metabolic acidosis. It is an acquired disorder of unknown aetiology.

Seventy to ninety percent of cases can be confirmed by palpating the abdomen for a small epigastric or right upper quadrant mobile ovoid mass (the "olive"). Visible gastric peristaltic waves may be seen going from left to right across the upper abdomen. Ultrasound or water-soluble contrast meal demonstrating the "string sign" will confirm the diagnosis.

cause of major gastrointestinal (GI) bleeding in teenagers. A further complication that a Meckel's can cause is a volvulus of the intestine if it is tethered to the abdominal wall. Occasionally it may also form the apex of an intussusception.

Very often the diagnosis of a Meckel's is made at laparotomy, but occasionally it may be possible to use a technetium scan in cases of intestinal bleeding to reveal a Meckel's by targeting the gastric mucosa within it. Once Meckel's diverticulum is identified, the treatment is simple — surgical excision.

TUMOURS OF THE SMALL INTESTINE

Tumours of the small intestine are relatively rare, comprising less than 5% of all GI tumours. Often examiners try to throw students off by asking about them. This is not because you are expected to know much about them but because it is a good question to ask to see if you can think and answer a question logically; for example, "Tell me about small bowel tumours."

Approach this sort of question as discussed in the chapter "Surgical Talk": small bowel tumours can be primary or secondary, benign or malignant.

Benign Tumours

These can arise from any of the elements of the bowel wall, such as the following:

- Lipomas (arise from fat)
- Leiomyomas (arise from smooth muscle)
- Neurofibromas (arise from nerves)
- Adenomas (arise from glandular mucosa)
- Adenomatous polyps of the small bowel may be premalignant (as in the colon). As with colonic adenomas, they may also be associated with polyposis syndromes and Peutz–Jeghers syndrome (pigmentation around the mouth and small bowel polyps). Benign tumours may either be found incidentally or present with bleeding or intussusception.

MALIGNANCY OF THE SMALL INTESTINE

Adenocarcinoma of the small intestine is occasionally seen and is believed in the majority of cases to arise from pre-existing adenomatous polyps (as in the colon). Lymphomas may also occur in the small bowel. Carcinoid tumours are of low-grade malignancy and are believed to arise from neuroectodermal cells embryologically. The commonest site for these is the appendix, but they can occur anywhere throughout the GI tract and are also found in the lung (bronchial carcinoids). These tumours release serotonin (5-HT) and kinins, which can cause symptoms if they get into the circulation. Normally these hormones are broken down by the liver in the first-pass metabolism from the gut and so no symptoms occur. However, in the presence of metastases there is no first-pass metabolism and the patient may suffer from carcinoid syndrome which consists of flushing, bronchospasm and diarrhoea.

INTUSSUSCEPTION

An intussusception can be defined as a condition where a portion of the intestine gets invaginated (by peristalsis) into its own lumen. The invaginated portion (the intussusceptum) can then be further propelled down the lumen for a variable distance.

A section through a piece of bowel containing an intussusception would contain two full layers of intestinal wall: the intussusceptum inside and the intussuscipiens outside (Figure 7.1).

Most intussusceptions are seen in children, usually infants under one year of age. They may present as colicky abdominal pain leading to obstruction. So-called redcurrant jelly stools may be passed (which consist of mucus and blood). The danger is that the intussusceptum may strangulate and infarct. Abdominal examination may reveal a mass and occasionally the apex of the intussusception may protrude from the anus or be felt on rectal examination.

In children, most intussusceptions are thought to be caused by peristalsis acting on a hypertrophied Peyer's patch. Meckel's diverticulum is another possible cause. Sometimes the intussusception can be reduced by a barium enema (so-called hydrostatic reduction), and if this is unsuccessful,

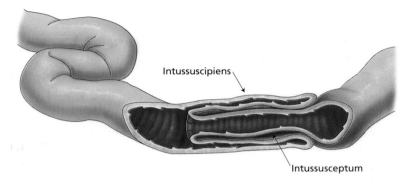

Figure 7.1.   Intussusception.

surgical correction is required. If possible the intussusception is simply reduced and recurrence is then uncommon. If it cannot be reduced or if it is non-viable, then the affected segment needs to be resected.

If intussusception occurs in an adult (which is rare), then a tumour (benign or malignant) acting as the apex of the intussusception should be considered and surgical resection of the involved segment with primary anastomosis is most often required.

ACUTE APPENDICITIS

Acute appendicitis is the commonest emergency surgical presentation requiring operation. Most cases are thought to be caused by obstruction of the appendix with subsequent infection behind the obstruction. This concept of an obstructed system getting infected is also relevant to conditions such as cholangitis (infection of an obstructed biliary tree) and pyonephrosis (infection of an obstructed renal tract). In appendicitis the most common cause of obstruction of the appendix is either a faecolith (a piece of faeces within the appendix) or hypertrophy of lymphoid tissue within the wall of the appendix, presumably in response to an otherwise minor viral infection. Rare causes of obstruction of the appendix and therefore appendicitis include carcinoma of the caecum and carcinoid tumour.

To understand the way in which appendicitis presents clinically, one should realise that in its early stages the inflammation of the appendix is confined to the wall of the appendix itself and is therefore felt as a poorly localised visceral pain in the central abdominal (originates in the embryological midgut). Because the essential feature is of an obstructed appendix, the pain will usually be colicky due to peristalsis in the appendicular muscle. As the inflammatory process progresses, the surrounding tissues and parietal peritoneum become inflamed and the pain is then felt locally in the right iliac fossa and is constant and typical of a localised peritonitis, worse on movement, etc. The typical patient will therefore present with an initial central colicky abdominal pain, which after a few hours progresses into a constant right iliac fossa pain (the pain moves; it does not radiate). By this time the patient will usually have a mild fever, be anorexic and may have nausea and vomiting. On examination there will be localised right iliac fossa tenderness and guarding with rebound tenderness or percussion tenderness. The diagnosis is essentially a clinical one and in straightforward cases no investigations at all are required.

The treatment of acute appendicitis is appendicectomy. It would be very reasonable of an examiner to ask simple questions about the operation, as it is the most common one performed as an emergency. For that reason the basic steps of an appendicectomy are outlined here.

Appendicectomy

First of all, an incision is made in the right iliac fossa. Conventionally this would be centred over McBurney's point, which is two-thirds of the way along a line drawn from the umbilicus to the anterior superior iliac spine. In practice, many surgeons make a slightly lower incision, which is cosmetically more acceptable. However, McBurney's point is often asked about in examinations because it marks the usual site of the base of the appendix. An incision is then made down through skin and subcutaneous tissues until the muscle layers are reached. The external oblique, internal oblique and transverse abdominis muscles are then opened. This is done by a muscle-splitting incision along the lines of the fibres with no fibres actually being cut. The final layer is the peritoneum, which is opened so that the abdominal cavity can be entered. The appendix and caecum are then identified and pulled up through the incision.

There seems to be a misconception among many medical students that the retrocaecal appendix is unusual. In fact this is the commonest site of the appendix. After delivery of the appendix the blood vessels and mesentery of the appendix are divided and the appendix is ligated and removed at its base. Many surgeons then bury the stump of the appendix with a purse-string suture around the caecum. The caecum is then returned to the abdomen. Any fluid or pus is carefully sucked and swabbed out. If there is severe contamination a drain may be left. The layers of the abdominal muscles are then closed using an absorbable suture.

The operation should be covered with prophylactic antibiotics, usually metronidazole, given intravenously at induction of the anaesthetic. Alternatively, diagnostic laparoscopy can be performed in these patients with laparoscopic appendicectomy where this is suspected or confirmed to be the source of inflammation.

Another misconception that many students (and indeed doctors) have relates to the presence of tenderness on rectal examination. Only 7% of appendixes lie in a pelvic position and most of these do not reach far enough into the pelvis to be in any way near to an examining finger. Therefore, when patients have rectal tenderness in association with acute appendicitis, it is not because of the adjacent position of the inflamed appendix; it is in fact because inflammatory fluids and perhaps pus have tracked down from the area of the appendix in the right iliac fossa to the most dependent portion of the abdominal cavity, the pouch of Douglas.

Occasionally, acute appendicitis may present after it has been fully walled off by the omentum and small bowel. At this stage (usually more than 72 h after the onset of symptoms) a mass is usually present on palpation. This may either resolve with antibiotics or develop into an abscess (which may be amenable to radiologically guided percutaneous drainage). Most surgeons would advocate an interval appendicectomy at about three months (Ochsner–Sherren regimen) on the basis that 20% of patients will develop recurrent appendicitis otherwise.

Causes of a Right Iliac Fossa Mass

- Appendix mass
- Gynaecological mass (e.g. ovarian cyst)

- Caecal cancer
- Soft tissue tumour (e.g. sarcoma)
- Lymph node mass
- Tuberculosis
- Actinomycosis
- Transplant kidney
- Iliac aneurysm

MESENTERIC ADENITIS

Mesenteric adenitis is the main differential diagnosis for acute appendicitis. It is a condition where enlargement of the mesenteric lymph nodes occurs, causing pain and a temperature, as well as local tenderness. It is mostly seen in children and adolescents and is often associated with a viral or upper respiratory tract infection. Headache and photophobia are more common than acute appendicitis. The temperature is often higher than in acute appendicitis and the tenderness and pain may not be as focal. Investigation shows lymphocytosis rather than a raised neutrophil count. No specific treatment other than paracetamol is usually required. If operative exploration is undertaken to rule out appendicitis then the appendix should be removed, whether or not it is normal, in order to avoid confusion over any subsequent attacks of abdominal pain.

SMALL BOWEL OBSTRUCTION

The commonest cause of small bowel obstruction in the Western world is adhesions, secondary to previous surgery, and the second commonest cause is hernias. Other causes can be classified as shown in Table 7.1.

The precise symptoms and presentation depend on the site of the obstruction, but the four cardinal features are as follows:

- Pain
- Abdominal distension
- Vomiting
- Absolute constipation

Table 7.1.   Causes of Intestinal Obstruction

In the lumen
> Impacted faeces or food bolus obstruction
> Swallowed foreign body
> Large polyps
> Intussusception

In the wall
> Tumours
> Infarction
> Crohn's disease
> Benign stricture

Outside the wall
> Adhesions
> Strangulated hernia
> Volvulus
> Extrinsic compression

The pain is usually colicky in nature, i.e. intermittent spasms of pain due to peristalsis which wear off after a few seconds, only to return a few minutes later. The pain is often severe and makes the patient double up whilst it is present. Pain due to small bowel obstruction is usually found in the central abdomen (embryological midgut). Distension is variable and depends on the level of the obstruction, with more distal obstructions causing greater degrees of distension, as one might expect. Likewise, vomiting occurs early with high intestinal obstruction and late with low intestinal obstruction. Absolute constipation means that the patient is passing neither flatus nor faeces. In high obstruction absolute constipation may not be present.

Abdominal examination may reveal distension and hyperactive bowel sounds. Focal tenderness implies that strangulation might be occurring. Strangulation refers to compromise of part of the intestinal blood supply due to twisting or kinking of its mesentery. It may also be suggested by findings of a temperature or raised white count and obviously in later stages will progress to gangrene and perforation of the bowel with signs of generalised peritonitis. A plain abdominal X-ray may be helpful in confirming the diagnosis of small bowel obstruction. The typical appearance would be of distended small bowel loops (remember that the small bowel usually has a diameter of less than 4 cm on a plain X-ray and is characterised by its central position within the abdomen and valvulae conniventes which go all the way across the bowel lumen).

Treatment of Small Bowel Obstruction

The patient should be carefully assessed and on abdominal examination particular attention should be paid to the presence of previous abdominal scars or the presence of hernias. The groin should be very carefully examined, as a small femoral hernia can be easily missed unless specifically looked for. If a hernia is found in a patient who is obstructed, then immediate surgery is required to repair the hernia and release the obstruction, as it is likely that the bowel is strangulated within the hernia.

At operation the bowel should be carefully inspected, and if it is thought to be non-viable a resection of that section of the bowel may be required. If the obstruction is thought to be due to adhesions and if there are no suggestions that strangulation has already occurred, then a period of conservative management may be appropriate. This usually consists of keeping the patient nil by mouth, passing a nasogastric tube (NGT) which should be left on free drainage with two-hourly aspiration in an attempt to decompress the bowel, and giving intravenous fluids to avoid dehydration ("drip and suck"). The patient should then be carefully monitored and the resolution of the obstruction would be marked by a lessening of pain, a decrease in the NGT aspirate volumes, the passage of flatus and the resolution of signs on a repeat X-ray. Should the patient not settle within 24 h or should signs of strangulation develop, then surgery would be indicated. Surgery for adhesions normally consists of a laparotomy at which the adhesions are divided.

The term "subacute bowel obstruction" is sometimes used to describe the condition where only one or two of the four cardinal signs are present. However, this term is really meaningless and obstruction should be classified as complete or partial. There is one other term used, "pseudo-obstruction". This means the patient is obstructed but no mechanical cause can be found. It may be due to many factors, such as electrolyte abnormalities, trauma or medications.

LARGE BOWEL OBSTRUCTION

The commonest causes of acute large bowel obstruction are carcinoma of the colon, diverticulitis and volvulus of the sigmoid or caecum. Unlike small bowel obstruction, adhesions and hernias are rarer causes. Like small bowel obstruction, large bowel obstruction gives rise to distension, colicky abdominal pain, vomiting and constipation; although the onset of vomiting may take longer. In 20% of people the ileocaecal valve is competent and decompression of the large bowel back into the small bowel cannot occur. This is a dangerous situation, as pressure can rapidly build up in the colon, leading to a perforation, which is the major complication in large bowel obstruction. Perforation usually occurs in the caecum, as this is the thinnest-walled and most distensible part of the colon. Investigations would be blood tests (full blood count (FBC), urea and electrolytes (U&E), amylase and group and save) and X-rays. Sigmoidoscopy may show the site of the lesion and an emergency contrast enema may be helpful in differentiating true obstruction from pseudo-obstruction.

Management is intravenous resuscitation and passage of a nasogastric tube. Immediate laparotomy is indicated if signs of peritonitis are present (indicating perforation has occurred) or if the caecum is greater than 10 cm in diameter or very tender, indicating imminent perforation. Recently, self-expanding metallic stents have proved useful in the treatment of large bowel obstruction. These stents can be inserted through the stricture under endoscopic or radiological guidance and are thus useful in the palliation of patients who are unfit for major surgery. They can also be useful to decompress acutely obstructing cancers and thus obviate the need for emergency surgery in an acutely unwell patient.

INFLAMMATORY BOWEL DISEASE

Inflammatory bowel disease is a term which includes both ulcerative colitis (UC) and Crohn's disease.

Crohn's Disease

Crohn's disease is a chronic, relapsing, transmural granulomatous disorder (i.e. on histology the whole thickness of the bowel is affected and granulomas are seen) of unknown aetiology. It can occur anywhere in the GI tract, from mouth to anus, but is commonest in the terminal ileum (hence its old name, "terminal ileitis"). It can affect the colon, where occasionally it may be difficult to differentiate from ulcerative colitis. It will often affect separate areas of the bowel with normal bowel in between (so-called "skip" lesions). It tends to produce healing by fibrosis, resulting in strictures, and has a tendency to form fistulae to other structures, such as adjacent loops of bowel, the bladder, the vagina and the skin surface.

The way in which Crohn's disease first presents varies with its site and extent. The commonest presentation will be with a change in the bowel habit, usually diarrhoea, central abdominal colicky pains or pains in the right iliac fossa, fever, anorexia, weight loss and general malaise. On examination there may be tenderness or a mass in the abdomen, most often in the right iliac fossa. Often, however, there are no abnormal physical signs. Investigation consists of the exclusion of other possible diagnoses, including carcinoma. Blood tests may be helpful and show elevated acute phase proteins, especially C-reactive protein. The mainstay of diagnosis, however, involves contrast studies (barium follow-through examination of the small bowel or barium enema for the colon) and endoscopic studies with biopsy (e.g. colonoscopy).

Most cases of Crohn's disease are initially managed medically by gastroenterologists, although about 65% will at some time require surgery. Drugs such as mesalazine and steroids may be used. Severe cases where there is stricture formation, fistulisation or an inflammatory mass that is not resolving may need surgical intervention.

The surgery for Crohn's disease depends on which part of the bowel is affected. The treatment can be divided into surgery for small and large bowel disease.

If the small bowel is predominantly involved, the main aims of surgery will be to perform strictureplasties or resect the very diseased bowel locally but to minimise resection as much as possible. The reason for this is that occasional patients may require repeated surgery and end up with short gut syndrome if too much bowel is resected. (The main concern in short gut syndrome is liquid stools, although patients also have vitamin and nutritional deficiencies.) In large bowel disease the operation usually performed is panproctocolectomy with ileostomy (removal of the whole large bowel and anus) or subtotal colectomy with ileorectal anastomosis (if the rectum is spared of disease). Smaller, more limited resections of the large bowel in Crohn's are associated with high relapse rates requiring further surgery.

Detailed questions about Crohn's disease are most likely to come from gastroenterologists in medical exams. However, you should obviously know about the associated complications outside the abdomen, including the high incidence of perianal disease such as abscesses and perianal fistulae, the skin changes of erythema nodosum and pyoderma gangraenosum, the associated arthritis and ocular problems.

Ulcerative Colitis (UC)

Unlike Crohn's disease, ulcerative colitis affects only the colon, and whilst Crohn's disease affects the full thickness of the bowel wall, ulcerative colitis affects only the mucosa. Another difference from Crohn's disease is that UC usually affects the rectum and as the disease gets more extensive it spreads proximally in a continual pattern (i.e. skip lesions should make one consider Crohn's disease). Like Crohn's disease, UC is a chronic and relapsing condition. The normal mode of presentation will be of blood-stained diarrhoea and abdominal pain, which is often eased by defaecation. (Note: UC tends to present with bloody diarrhoea whereas Crohn's tends to present with painful diarrhoea.) In most cases there are no abnormal physical signs. In more severe cases, nausea, vomiting and distension may occur in association with pyrexia, and this should make one suspect the development of toxic megacolon.

In non-acute cases investigation consists of the elimination of other pathologies, and confirmation is usually made by biopsy on sigmoidoscopy or colonoscopy. It can sometimes be difficult for the histologist to differentiate Crohn's from UC, and may call the condition as "indeterminate" or non-specific inflammatory bowel disease. The other major difference between Crohn's disease and UC is that while the former appears to have only a small premalignant potential, the latter is most definitely premalignant. The figure usually quoted is that for ulcerative colitis involving most of the colon there is a 10% risk of developing a carcinoma for every ten years that the disease exists. Because of this, people with UC are advised to have regular routine screening colonoscopies with biopsies every 2–3 years. The particular feature looked for on the biopsy is the development of dysplasia, and if it is severe, consideration should be given to the possibility of an elective total colectomy to reduce the risk of cancer formation.

The operation will normally be a proctocolectomy, which means that the whole of the colon and rectum will be removed so that no colonic mucosa will be left. After this the patient either is left with a terminal ileostomy or can have a new pelvic reservoir (a pouch) constructed, which is made by joining several loops of small bowel together and sewing that directly down to the anal sphincters. A pouch operation would nowadays normally be offered to any person requiring a total colectomy for UC. Such an operation cannot be offered to patients with Crohn's colitis, because Crohn's disease often recurs in the small bowel used to construct the reservoir and the results of the operation are therefore poor.

The majority of UC patients (>85%) can be managed medically (antidiarrhoeals, steroids, mesalazine, etc.), unlike Crohn's disease, in which about 65% will require surgery at some point. The principal acute complication of UC which you need to know about and which might require surgical intervention is toxic megacolon. This is diagnosed on a plain X-ray and is defined as dilatation of the transverse colon above 6 cm. The patient will normally be quite unwell with UC and will present with severe blood-stained diarrhoea and systemic signs such as fever, dehydration and tachycardia. There is usually abdominal tenderness and the white cell count may be raised. Initial attempts will usually be made to treat the patient conservatively with intravenous fluids, correction of electrolyte abnormalities and high-dose intravenous steroids. Repeated abdominal X-rays should be taken to watch the size of the colon (usually the transverse colon), and if it appears to be getting bigger despite appropriate medical treatment, an operation is indicated before it perforates. Also, if a perforation is suspected or if the patient fails to settle within 24–48 h of medical treatment, then surgery will be indicated.

In this situation the usual surgical procedure is a total colectomy, an ileostomy and the rectal stump is usually oversewn or brought out to the skin so that it can be inspected (this is called a mucous fistula). Subsequently, when the acute problem has settled, the patient could be offered an ileal reservoir or completion proctectomy (i.e. removal of the rest of the rectum and anus, leaving the patient with a permanent ileostomy) according to discussions between the surgeon and patient.

It is not uncommon to be shown a barium enema during your viva, and the commonest diagnoses are ulcerative colitis or an apple core stricture indicating malignancy. You may also be shown a barium meal with follow-through which looks at the small bowel (you see some contrast in the stomach and hence you can tell it is a follow-through), and this may show the strictures of Crohn's disease.

COLON CANCER

Colon cancer is the commonest GI cancer and questions are therefore common in surgical finals. Patients who have had previous operations for colon cancer are often brought up as long cases. The way in which colon cancer presents depends partly on its position within the colon. Tumours on the right side of the colon are more likely to present later with a mass or anaemia, since the faeces are still liquid in this region and thus are less likely to produce an obstruction to the flow. In contradistinction, tumours on the left side of the colon are more likely to present early with obstruction and a change in bowel habit. Tumours in the rectum may give rise to tenesmus, which is a symptom where the patient feels as though there are some faeces which they need to pass even after they have just emptied their bowels. This symptom is actually a reflection of the mass present within the rectum. Examination may be entirely normal. Rectal examination is mandatory, as you may be able to feel a low rectal tumour. Sigmoidoscopy should also be performed, which will allow visualisation (and biopsy) of tumours in the last 15 cm or so of the intestinal tract (which may be missed on barium enema). Investigations — simple blood tests (FBC, U&E, LFTs) and carcinoembryonic antigen (CEA, a marker for bowel cancer) — should be measured. Further investigation is usually with barium enema (apple core lesion) or colonoscopy, where a stricture or mass will be found. Colonoscopy allows biopsies to be taken. A computed tomography (CT) scan is performed to stage and screen for liver metastases.

A common question relates to the staging of colon cancer. The classical way of staging such tumours is Dukes' staging. Initially Sir Cuthbert Dukes (a pathologist at St Mark's Hospital, London) described three stages: A, where the tumour is confined to the mucosa and submucosa of the bowel wall (this has a 90% five-year survival rate); B, where the tumour has invaded into or through the bowel wall into surrounding tissue but the lymph nodes are clear (this has a 60% five-year survival rate); C, where the lymph nodes are involved. Stage C is usually divided into C1 and C2. C2 is where the highest lymph node in the surgical specimen is involved (implying further spread). Overall, Stage C has a five-year survival of about 30%. Although not originally described by Dukes, the further Stage D is now usually mentioned where there is distant spread, and this has a 5–10% five-year survival rate.

Dukes' staging system has been largely superseded by the TNM classification system where T refers to the depth of tumour invasion, N refers to lymph node involvement and M refers to the presence of metastatic disease. The treatment of colon cancer is surgery and resection of the tumour. Tumours of the right colon usually undergo right hemicolectomy, tumours of the transverse colon undergo an extended right hemicolectomy, and the descending colon tumours undergo left hemicolectomy. When resecting bowel cancers, attention is paid to the blood supply to the segment involved. There must be a good blood supply to the two cut ends; therefore, the surgeon removes the entire part of the bowel supplied by the blood vessels supplying the tumour (and hence are ligated when the tumour is resected). Thus a tumour of the caecum (supplied by the right colic artery) means a right hemicolectomy.

Tumours of the rectum are treated by anterior resection (where the rectal tumour is removed and the colon above the tumour is anastomosed to the remaining rectal stump). Usually a primary anastomosis is performed using either sutures or a staple gun. If the anastomosis is formed at the pelvic floor following total mesorectal excision (TME), then a proximal temporary stoma (usually an ileostomy) is usually constructed and closed a few weeks later. This is in order to divert the faeces away from the healing anastomosis. If the tumour is very low down and excision cannot be performed without involving the anal sphincters, then an abdominoperineal (AP) resection (i.e. excision of the rectum and anus) is required. This is a much more extensive operation and leaves the patient with two wounds (the perineal and the laparotomy) and a permanent end colostomy.

In terms of the latest developments in the understanding of rectal cancer, it is now thought that the presence of radial spread (in an outward direction from the bowel into the surrounding mesentery) is an important prognostic indicator. Therefore many surgeons nowadays perform a careful total mesorectal excision (removing the mesentery of the rectum) during an anterior resection in order to reduce the incidence of local recurrence. Laparoscopic surgery for the removal of colorectal cancer has been shown in several international multicentre randomised trials to offer superior short-term recovery and equivalent long-term oncological outcomes, and is now recommended to be offered as an alternative to open surgical resection for suitable tumours (excluding some T4 tumours) provided that the operating surgeon has been adequately trained.

The role of adjuvant therapy in colorectal cancer is still unclear. Many studies have been published and many more are still underway. At present it appears that systemic chemotherapy with 5-fluorouracil and levamisole leads to increased survival and decreased recurrence in patients with Dukes' C cancers. The role of chemotherapy in Dukes' B cancers is less clear. Radiotherapy is of no value in colon cancer (as the tumour is too mobile and not particularly radiosensitive) but has been shown to be associated with improved outcome in some patients with rectal cancer if given preoperatively over a short (five days) or long (five weeks) course.

Stomas and Types of Colonic Resections

Questions on these are common. The following is a simple guide. A stoma in the right lower quadrant is usually an ileostomy. Because small bowel content is an irritant to the skin, ileostomies are usually constructed with a spout and they stand clear of the skin by a few centimetres. They may be either an end ileostomy in someone who has had a total colectomy or a loop ileostomy where the bowel has been temporarily defunctioned. The latter type is usually performed after a total mesorectal excision to give the anastomosis time to heal before restoring intestinal continuity. Obviously, the end ileostomy will have only one opening whilst the loop ileostomy will have two. However, students will not usually be expected to remove ileostomy bags to confirm this in exams. There can be large fluid losses from an ileostomy, particularly in the initial stages, and it is important to regularly measure the losses and replace them accordingly via a drip to prevent dehydration.

A stoma in the right upper quadrant is usually a defunctioning transverse colostomy. Like the defunctioning ileostomy, it will have two lumens, but will not usually have a spout and is therefore flush with the skin surface. Again it will usually be a temporary stoma to cover an anastomosis.

Stomas are not usually constructed in the left upper quadrant; however, if there is one it is probably one of the types found in the left lower quadrant, which for technical reasons has been sited higher than usual.

Left lower quadrant stomas may be either end colostomies, loop colostomies or double-barrelled colostomies. An end colostomy is produced after resection of the rectum or sigmoid colon (Figure 7.2). There is an operation called Hartmann's procedure, in which the sigmoid colon is resected and the rectal stump is left inside the pelvis and closed with sutures, while a temporary end colostomy is brought out in the left lower quadrant. This is most often performed for perforated diverticulitis, where the affected portion of the bowel is resected but the contamination makes it unsafe to join the ends back together immediately. A permanent end colostomy is produced after complete excision of the anus and rectum (an abdominoperineal excision) for a very low rectal cancer. If after a resection it is thought unsafe to join the bowel ends together, but the distal end is long enough, then both ends may be brought out together to the surface. This is called a double-barrelled colostomy (Figure 7.3). If the bowel is long enough, it is preferred to a Hartmann's, because reversal does not require a full relaparotomy. Loop colostomy is when the apex of the sigmoid is brought out as a stoma without a resection having been performed. This is occasionally done for an inoperable carcinoma of the rectum that is likely to obstruct.

Screening for Colorectal Cancer

Colonoscopy is the ideal test but is expensive. The haemoccult test, which looks for faecal occult blood (FOB), is one of the better and cheaper tests. However, it has a relatively low sensitivity and gives a high

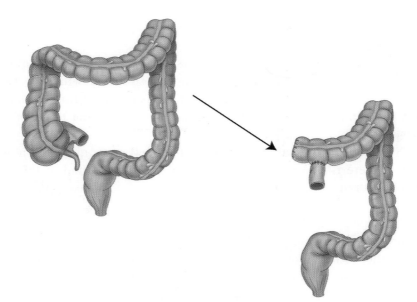

Figure 7.2(a).   Colonic resections: right hemicolectomy.

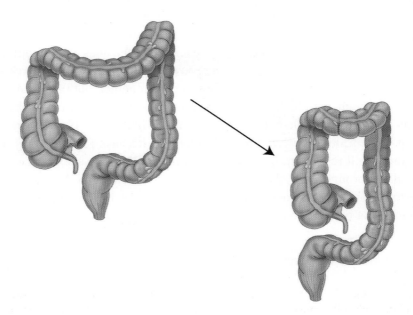

Figure 7.2(b).   Colonic resections: transverse colectomy.

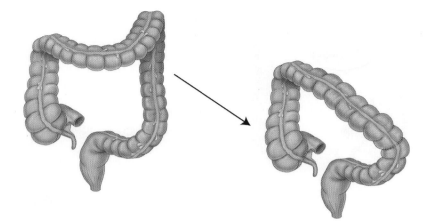

Figure 7.2(c).   Colonic resections: left hemicolectomy.

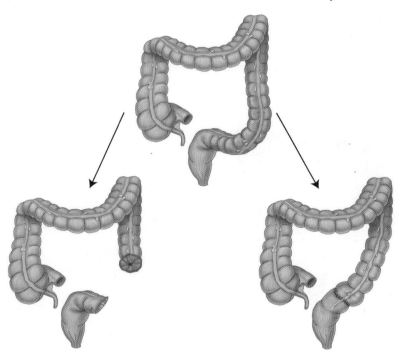

Figure 7.2(d).   Colonic resections: surgery for disease of the sigmoid colon or rectum —
(i) Hartmann's, (ii) sigmoid colectomy. The decision about which operation is performed
depends on several factors, including the disease process, the skill of the surgeon and the
general health of the patient.

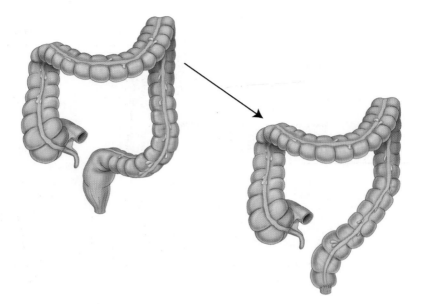

Figure 7.2(e).   Colonic resections: anterior resection.

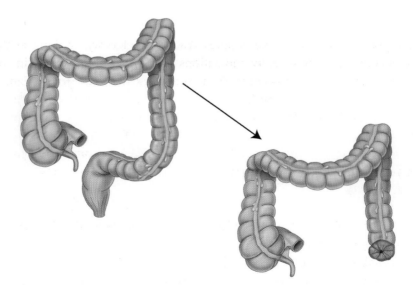

Figure 7.2(f).   Colonic resections: abdominoperineal resection (note that there are two wounds — the laparotomy and the perineal wound — and a stoma).

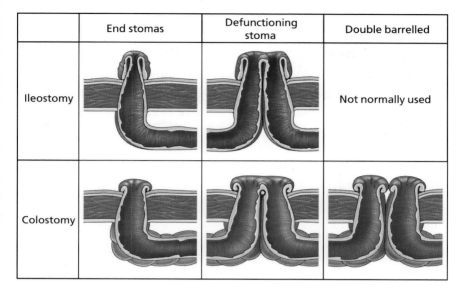

	End stomas	Defunctioning stoma	Double barrelled
Ileostomy			Not normally used
Colostomy			

Figure 7.3. The different types of stomas. In the double-barrelled colostomy the distal end is sometimes known as a mucous fistula. This allows it to be inspected and reversal, if necessary, is easier.

false positive rate. Even so, studies that are underway, looking at the haemoccult test, show early indications of decreased mortality in the screened groups. This has led to the setting up of the NHS Bowel Cancer Screening Programme which uses FOB to screen the population aged 60–69 years. This is followed by colonoscopy for those who screen positive for FOB.

In addition to those screened as part of the NHS national programme, consideration should also be given to screening the following high-risk groups:

- Those with familial adenomatous polyposis (who usually have a colectomy early)
- Strong family history (more than two close relatives)
- Anyone with a personal history of polyps or colorectal cancer
- Patients with pancolitis for more than ten years, Peutz–Jeghers, juvenile polyposis, etc.

Carcinoembryonic antigen is a serological marker for colorectal cancer. However, it is not usually elevated in early disease (less than 5% of Dukes' A cancers have a raised CEA) and it also has low specificity, being raised in many other conditions (such as other inflammatory conditions of the GI tract, smoking or renal impairment). Therefore, it has little value in any screening programme. It is, however, used in the follow-up of patients with colorectal cancer. The level of CEA should fall to normal limits within weeks of the operation to remove the cancer. At the follow-up clinics, a rise in CEA can be used to diagnose recurrence of the tumour, often before it is clinically apparent.

Colonic Polyps

A polyp is defined as a lesion which projects into the lumen of the bowel. The relevance in the colon is mainly because of the tendency of some types of polyps to become malignant. The general term "polyp", however, is purely a morphological term and in no way defines the actual diagnosis for which histology would usually be required (most often obtained by biopsy or polypectomy at sigmoidoscopy or colonoscopy). It is helpful to consider polyps under their different pathological headings.

Adenomatous Polyps

Adenomatous polyps are important because of their tendency to lead to colorectal cancer. Most authorities believe that the majority of adenocarcinomas of the colon develop from pre-existing adenomatous polyps. Evidence for this belief includes the fact that early stages of malignancy (severe dysplasia and carcinoma *in situ*) may sometimes be found in polyps and that patients with familial adenomatous polyposis die of cancer at a young age unless they have a prophylactic colectomy. In addition, carcinogens which produce adenomas experimentally also lead to cancer formation, and studies in which patients were followed up after previous colorectal cancer, where polyps were prophylactically removed at colonoscopy, appeared to have a reduced incidence of subsequent new cancer development. The likelihood of an adenomatous polyp becoming malignant seems to relate to its size. It appears to be rare for adenomas under 1 cm in size but occurs with increasing likelihood as the polyp gets bigger. Adenomatous polyps of the colon are usually subclassified into the better-differentiated tubular adenomas (75%), which are often on a stalk, and the less-differentiated villous adenomas (10%), which are often sessile (i.e. flat). Sometimes a polyp is described as tubulovillous (15%) when it has an appearance somewhere between these two extremes.

Adenomas can be sporadic or familial. The familial adenomas occur in conditions such as familial multiple polyposis coli and Gardner's syndrome, and they have a high if not inevitable chance of developing into cancer.

Familial multiple polyposis coli is an autosomal dominant condition with multiple neoplastic colonic polyps beginning in the second to third decade, and patients usually have a prophylactic colectomy in their early 20s.

Gardner's syndrome is an autosomal dominant condition with multiple colonic adenomas in association with bony osteomas and epidermoid cysts.

Other than being premalignant, adenomatous polyps may present as follows:

- Bleeding which may be either frank blood or microscopic bleeding (present with anaemia).
- Polyps rarely present with a change in bowel habit, but a large benign polyp in the rectum can produce the symptoms of tenesmus (i.e. a sensation of incomplete evacuation due to the presence of a mass within the rectum).
- Some polyps may also secrete a large amount of mucus and the patient may complain of passing slime or jelly.
- Rarely, a polyp will prolapse through the anus or act as the apex for an intussusception.

Polyps may be diagnosed on imaging the colon with a barium enema, but if suspected the best investigation is usually a colonoscopy which gives the additional advantage of providing the opportunity for biopsy or complete removal of the polyp. Key points on histology, other than the diagnosis of an adenomatous polyp, will be whether or not there is any evidence of dysplasia of the cells on the surface of the polyp. Most histologists would classify this as mild, moderate or severe, with severe dysplasia being strongly suggestive that the lesion is premalignant.

Hamartomatous Polyps

A hamartoma (a lesion where there is an overgrowth of one or more of the cell types which are normal constituents of the organ from which they arise) is an unusual lesion defined as an abnormality of development. With regard to colonic polyps, there are two conditions in which hamartomatous polyps are normally described:

- *Juvenile polyps.* These have a low malignant potential. They may present with bleeding or intussusception and sometimes slough off spontaneously and actually present with material passed in the motion and noticed by the patient or parents. Usually it is possible to deal with them colonoscopically.
- *Peutz–Jeghers syndrome.* This is a rare autosomal dominant condition where multiple hamartomatous polyps appear throughout the entire GI tract. The affected individuals also have pigmentation of the skin around the lips and gums. Again the malignant potential of these polyps is small, although overall the patient is at a greater risk of developing carcinoma (both GI and non-GI tract).

Polyps Due to Protrusions of Mesenchymal Tissue

Conditions such as lipomas (benign tumours of fat), leiomyomas (benign tumours of smooth muscle), neurofibromas (benign tumours arising from nerve tissue) and haemangiomas (benign tumours of blood vessel origin) can all occur in the wall of the colon. If they then form a lump which protrudes into the lesion, they are by definition polyps. These are all rather rare in clinical practice and their main importance is that they may mimic the presentation of a carcinoma.

Metaplastic Polyps

These are sometimes also called hyperplastic polyps. They are usually small, often multiple and slightly raised above the surrounding normal mucosa. They have a distinctive histological appearance and have no malignant potential whatsoever. Because of their small size they cause no symptoms and their only relevance is in distinguishing them from adenomatous polyps. They are often seen in inflammatory bowel disease or lymphoid hyperplasia (such as at the appendix). If they are found incidentally at appendicectomy, then usually no other treatment is required.

Inflammatory Polyps

Examples are those found in inflammatory conditions of the bowel, such as pseudopolyps in ulcerative colitis.

DIVERTICULAR DISEASE

Diverticula are defined as outpouchings from a tubular structure (the opposite of polyps) (Figure 7.4). Colonic diverticula occur where the colonic mucosa bulges out at the weakest point where blood vessels enter the colonic muscle. They tend to appear in middle and old age and are much more common in Western countries, which may be due to the lack of fibre in the diet leading to muscle spasm and hence increased intraluminal pressure and bulging out of the mucosa. They are usually found on the left side of the colon, although they can occasionally involve all of the colon around as far as the caecum. They are extremely common, being found in the majority of elderly patients, especially if there is a history of constipation. Many are asymptomatic, but diverticular disease can be responsible for a number of clinical problems:

- Chronic symptoms of *gripey abdominal pains*, diarrhoea and passage of pellety stools are often ascribed to diverticular disease. Normal treatment is usually with antispasmodics and a high-fibre diet.
- *Acute diverticulitis*. This is a condition where a diverticulum becomes inflamed, usually because of the presence of inspissated faeces within it. In many ways it is similar to the process involved in acute appendicitis, and indeed diverticulitis is sometimes called left-sided appendicitis. The typical presentation would be an elderly patient, perhaps with a previous history of problems with constipation, etc., who presents with pain and tenderness in the left iliac fossa, a fever, local signs of peritonitis and a raised white cell count. The majority of

- Infective or ischaemic colitis
- Polyps
- Anal fissure
- Ulcerative colitis

The age of the patient is important — for example, haemorrhoids, cancer, diverticular disease and angiodysplasia are the most common in elderly patients, whereas infective colitis and ulcerative colitis are more common in young people.

In the history note the frequency and amount of bleeding, the colour (bright red blood is suggestive of lower GI bleeding, whereas dark red blood could be either upper or lower GI bleeding), whether the bleeding was associated with the passage of faeces and if so whether it was mixed in, whether there was any mucus or slime and whether there was any abdominal pain (suggestive of inflammatory disease). Examination should always include a proctoscopy (and if possible a rigid sigmoidoscopy) to look for a local cause of bleeding (e.g. haemorrhoids).

Resuscitation is the same as that for an upper GI bleed, although many cases stop bleeding spontaneously. If this is the case and there was a significant bleed, then the patient is admitted for urgent investigation. If the bleed is small and stops spontaneously, then the patient may be able to be investigated colonoscopically as an outpatient. Very occasionally the bleeding continues and is rapid, requiring an urgent angiogram to find the source of the bleeding. If a region of the bowel is shown to have abnormal blood vessels (i.e. angiodysplasia), then surgery to remove the affected area may be required (occasionally the bleeding vessel can be stopped by embolising the vessel radiologically). The operation required will depend on where the cause of the bleeding is.

In many cases it is impossible to tell from the history whether the bleed was from the upper or the lower GI tract, and in these cases the patient needs a gastroscopy initially to rule out an upper GI lesion.

8

RECTUM AND ANUS

Alan Horgan

MINOR ANO-RECTAL CONDITIONS

Haemorrhoids

There is much debate in surgical circles about the true nature of haemorrhoids. Unfortunately this sometimes manifests itself in finals as questions like "What exactly are haemorrhoids?" They are probably a vascular cushion, covered in a layer of mucosa and containing a branch of the superior rectal artery and a tributary of the superior rectal vein. The key point that the examiners will want you to make is that haemorrhoids are not simply dilated veins (when they bleed the blood is bright red). Haemorrhoids occur at the point where the superior rectal branches enter the muscle. Conventionally their position is described in relation to the anus imagined as a clock face visualised with the patient in the lithotomy position (i.e. on their back, with their legs up in stirrups). In this position the penis or vagina is anterior at 12 o'clock. There are usually three haemorrhoids, at 3, 7 and 11 o'clock.

Haemorrhoids are classified as follows:

- First degree: They do not prolapse from the anus
- Second degree: They prolapse on defaecation or straining but return spontaneously
- Third degree: They prolapse and remain prolapsed unless manually repositioned

Haemorrhoids may be asymptomatic, although if they do cause symptoms this is usually bleeding or minor pain and itching. They are usually not severely painful unless they are prolapsed and thrombosed. Bleeding from haemorrhoids is usually bright red and either on the outside of the motion or on the toilet paper. There is usually no change in the fundamental bowel habit and no other gastrointestinal symptoms or signs. Haemorrhoids can be treated by injection (with 5% phenol in almond oil); this works by shrinking the haemorrhoid through causing scar formation, by rubber band ligation or by coagulation with infrared devices. These procedures are usually performed in the outpatient department. If these methods fail, then it may be necessary to formally excise the haemorrhoids (haemorrhoidectomy), as a day case or an inpatient procedure.

Fissure *In Ano*

A fissure *in ano* usually starts with a tear in the anal canal caused by trauma or the passage of a constipated stool. In some cases this fails to heal and the inflammation it produces causes spasm of the sphincter muscle so that further trauma occurs when motions are passed and it eventually becomes a chronic fissure. Examination is often painful and it may be possible to see an external hypertrophic skin tag or sentinel pile, which is indurated at the base where the fissure lies.

The initial treatment for a fissure is conservative, with advice to avoid straining on the toilet (and the use of bulk laxatives) and the topical application of local anaesthetic gels. A variety of agents have recently been developed in order to promote relaxation of the internal anal sphincter. These include the use of topical nitrates (0.2% GTN paste), calcium channel blockers (2% diltiazem cream) and the injection of botulinum toxin into the internal anal sphincter. In the event of failure of the above conservative methods, then surgery may be needed. In the past the surgical treatment was manual dilatation of the anus under a general anaesthetic, but this was associated with high rates of long-term incontinence. Nowadays, chronic fissure is usually treated by the operation of lateral subcutaneous sphincterotomy, in which the external sphincter is partially divided through a small laterally placed stab incision.

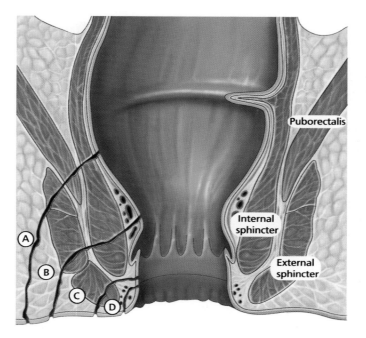

Figure 8.1.   Perianal fistulae. Cross-section through the anal canal and lower rectum showing the normal anatomy on the right and the different types of fistulae on the left: (A) pelvianal fistula, (B) high anal fistula, (C) low anal fistula, (D) subcutaneous anal fistula.

Fistula *In Ano*

A fistula is an abnormal connection between two epithelial surfaces. (Note: A sinus is a blind-ending tract joining an epithelial surface to a cavity lined by granulation tissue, e.g. an abscess.)

A fistula *in ano* has an opening internally to the anal canal and another opening externally onto the skin. Most probably start as a perianal abscess, but occasionally they are due to Crohn's disease, carcinoma, radiotherapy or tuberculosis. They can be classified as "low" when they do not cross the sphincter muscles above the dentate line and "high" when they cross the sphincters above this level (Figure 8.1). Low fistulae are usually treated by being laid open. This is achieved by inserting a metal probe into the fistula and incising through the tissue down onto the probe. The wound is allowed to heal from its depths upwards. This cannot be

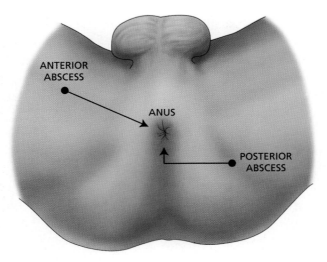

Figure 8.2.   Goodsall's rule.

done with high fistulae, because the sphincters would be damaged, and so these fistulae may be treated with a seton. This is a thread which is passed through the fistula track and is tied on the outside. It can then be gradually tightened so that over a period of weeks it cuts through to the surface, with the fistula healing by scar tissue behind it.

Goodsall's rule states that fistulae anterior to the anus usually open to the anus in a straight line whilst posterior ones usually have a curving track and open in the midline posteriorly (Figure 8.2).

Rectal Prolapse

Rectal prolapse may be partial or complete. Partial prolapse is defined as involving the mucosa alone and obviously this rarely prolapses for more than a few centimetres. Complete prolapse involves prolapse of the full thickness of the rectum and can be much more sizable. It is most common in elderly females and presents with a mass that appears on or during defaecation. It may reduce spontaneously or require manual reduction and sometimes will present as a semi-emergency as a prolapse which has become oedematous and ulcerated, producing pain and bleeding.

Rectal prolapse is usually associated with poor anal sphincter function. Initial treatment is to reduce the prolapse manually, but this will often be only a temporary solution. Partial-thickness (mucosal) prolapse may be treated by phenol injection (to induce scarring), rubber band ligation or by simple excision of the mucosa with plication of the underlying tissues (Delorme's procedure). Full-thickness prolapse usually needs surgical intervention such as an abdominal rectopexy (where the abdomen is entered and the rectum is stitched up, usually onto the sacrum, in order to prevent further prolapse). This can usually be performed laparoscopically with or without the use of mesh to fix the rectum to the presacral fascia. For those patients who may not be fit enough for abdominal surgery, then a perineal approach (Delorme's procedure or perineal rectosigmoidectomy) has less morbidity but higher rates of recurrence.

Perianal Haematoma

A perianal haematoma is sometimes also called a thrombosed external haemorrhoid (which is a misnomer, as it is not actually a haemorrhoid). It is usually due to subcutaneous bleeding around the anal margin caused by the passage of constipated stool. It produces acute perianal pain which may be worsened by defaecation or movement. Examination will reveal a tense, tender, blue lump at the anal margin which can be simply treated by incision under local anaesthetic should the symptoms be too severe to be controlled by simple analgesia. This may not be possible if the patient presents more than 24–48 h after the onset of symptoms, and therefore surgical excision under local or general anaesthesia may be necessary.

Anorectal Abscess

Anorectal or perianal abscesses are common problems and are frequently seen as emergencies. They may either be perianal, ischiorectal or intermuscular (where they extend between the internal and external sphincters) (Figure 8.3). Occasionally they represent spread from a pelvic abscess down to the perianal region. It is thought that there are two main reasons for the development of these abscesses. First, they may develop from anal gland infections. These will usually have intestinal-type organisms within

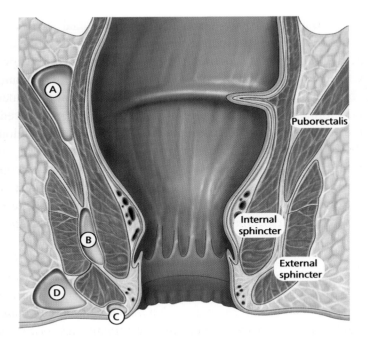

Figure 8.3.   Perianal abscesses: (A) pelvirectal abscess, (B) intersphinteric abscess, (C) perianal abscess, (D) ischiorectal abscess.

them (e.g. *Escherichia coli*). Others may develop from simple skin infections, such as an infected sebaceous gland or hair follicle, and are therefore more likely to contain *Staphylococci*.

The patient will usually be complaining of a severe throbbing pain, which is worse on sitting, and may have signs of a fever, tachycardia, etc. The treatment is surgical drainage, packing and healing by secondary intention. The patient should be seen subsequently in the outpatient clinic to see if there is any evidence of an underlying fistula *in ano*, which occurs in up to 30% of patients.

Pilonidal Abscess/Sinus

The word "pilonidal" comes from a Latin word meaning "nest of hair". A pilonidal abscess or sinus is usually found in the natal cleft. The exact aetiology is still not completely understood but it is thought to be an acquired rather than a congenital (as was once thought) condition. The hairs within the pilonidal cavity are thought to be hairs which have worked their way under the skin and not hairs growing within the sinus or abscess cavity. The condition is more common in people in their teenage and young adult years. It is more common in men than in women and, as one might expect, in those who are particularly hairy. It also seems to be more common in those whose occupation involves prolonged sitting, such as those who drive for a living.

The patient is usually unaware of the sinus until it becomes secondarily infected and presents as an abscess. Treatment of a pilonidal abscess is incision and drainage, followed by packing and healing by secondary intention. Later on, a second procedure is needed to excise the sinus tract (which may extend for some distance away from the opening and which can be outlined by injection of methylene blue into the orifices of the sinuses at the time of surgery). If the excised area is small enough it may be possible to close the area primarily. Alternatively it may be necessary to leave the area open to heal by secondary intention. Pilonidal disease has a significant tendency to recur even after apparently successful surgery. Patients should be encouraged to be scrupulous with their personal hygiene and to keep the area clean and dry and free from any loose hairs.

9

THE ACUTE ABDOMEN

Jeremy French

It is unlikely that any cases of acute abdominal pain will be seen as clinical cases in the finals. However, cases who have had previous acute abdominal problems may be included as clinical cases and questions on acute abdominal conditions are commonly found in MCQs or discussed in vivas. Indeed, examiners often place great importance on candidates having a good knowledge of the diagnosis and management of the acute abdomen, as they know that the subject will be of immediate relevance when the candidate takes up their general surgical foundation year job. The acute abdomen is commonly defined as a case of abdominal pain with a short history (usually less than one week), presenting as an emergency with no history of trauma. It is worth remembering, when answering questions, that such patients will usually be assessed in casualty departments or dedicated receiving wards and, as well as history and examination, simple investigations such as blood tests and plain X-rays are likely to be all that is initially available. To a large extent the management of the acute abdomen is not, therefore, based on complex investigations but on clinical acumen.

ABDOMINAL PAIN

As with all pains, a certain number of features should be elicited, namely:

- Site (at onset and currently) (see Figure 9.1).
- What is the nature of the pain (character, frequency, radiation)?
- How did the pain start and what has happened to it since?

163

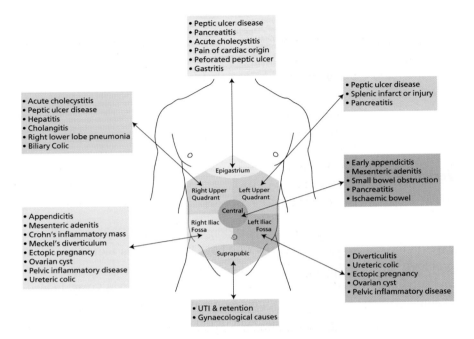

Figure 9.1.   Areas of the abdomen. The boxes contain the possible diagnoses of pain in these regions.

- What relieves and what exacerbates the pain?
- Are there any associated symptoms?
- Have you ever had this before?/Previous history.
- What do you think it is?

It is helpful to consider the underlying aetiology of the pain so as to try and classify types of acute abdominal pain further. In broad terms, pain in the acute abdomen is caused by one of the following:

- Visceral (organ) pain
  - Stimulation of the visceral peritoneum
  - Obstruction of a hollow viscus
- Parietal pain: Inflammation of the parietal peritoneum (i.e. peritonitis)
- Referred pain (e.g. pain referred from nerve root compression)

Colic is defined as pain caused by obstruction of a hollow viscus and, in the context of the acute abdomen, may arise from obstruction of the small intestine, ureter, biliary system, colon, uterus, fallopian tubes or appendix. When a hollow viscus with smooth muscle in its walls is obstructed, the smooth muscle contracts in peristaltic waves in an attempt to overcome the obstruction. These spasmodic contractions give rise to intermittent spasms of pain. The classical example is small bowel colic, where pain will come and grip the patient for a short period of time, be so severe as to double them up or make them cry out with pain, and then wear off before another attack occurs, usually a few minutes later. Visceral pain is usually not well localised and probably travels along the autonomic nerves which have no dermatomal distribution.

The gut develops embryologically from midline structures and hence pain is generally referred to the midline. Foregut structures (lower third of the oesophagus to the ampulla of Vater in the second part of the duodenum) usually give rise to pain in the epigastrium, midgut structures (second part of the duodenum to two thirds along the transverse colon) give rise to pain in the periumbilical region, and hindgut structures (ending at the proximal rectum) give rise to pain in the suprapubic region. Thus small bowel colic is usually felt periumbilically, etc.

Parietal pain is caused by stimulation of the visceral peritoneum, which covers the intra-abdominal organs (e.g. hepatic capsular stretch by tumour, or splenic capsular stimulation due to infarction). Inflammation of this structure is called peritonitis. In contrast to the viscera, the parietal peritoneum is innervated by somatic nerves and hence pain is accurately localised to the site of inflammation. This type of pain is typically worse with movement, coughing or inspiration and therefore the patient lies still with shallow breaths (unlike colicky pain, where they move about to try to get comfortable).

Peritonitis is associated with guarding or rigidity of the abdominal muscles. There appears to be some difference in opinion as to the true definition of guarding and rigidity; however, most surgeons would agree that guarding is an involuntary (reflex) contraction of the abdominal muscles when the examining hand presses down over the inflamed area. It is sometimes difficult to differentiate true guarding from voluntary guarding, where the patient contracts their own abdominal muscles in anticipation of pain (especially seen in children). However, if you palpate the two sides of the abdomen at the same time while distracting the patient, you may find that the muscles appear tense on one side compared to the other. It is not really possible to do this voluntarily (where the two sides contract symmetrically) and hence this must be true guarding. If at rest the patient's abdominal musculature has an increased tone, then this is termed rigidity and is again due to underlying inflammation of the peritoneum. If peritonitis involves the whole abdomen, then the patient would typically present with a board-like, rigid, tender abdomen with absent bowel sounds.

EXAMINATION OF THE ABDOMEN

It is always important to do a general examination of the patient, in particular, paying attention to signs of shock or dehydration as manifested by peripheral shutdown, clamminess, pallor, tachypnoea, tachycardia and hypotension. One can often tell, just by looking at the patient, whether they are unwell. The typical patient with peritonitis looks pale and sweaty, with sunken eyes and a weak thready pulse, shallow breaths and little movement — as first described by Hippocrates thousands of years ago.

Introduce yourself to the patient; ask if they mind your examination and if they have any pain. Lay the patient flat (one pillow) and adequately undress them (ideally from the nipples to the knees, but in the exam you should try to preserve the patient's dignity). On inspection of the abdomen (from the foot of the bed) observe for any obvious scars or masses, drains, dressings or stomas, distension and the movement with respiration. The common surgical scars that you may encounter can be seen in Figure 9.2. You may find it easier in an exam situation to comment on your observations as you go along (unless you are confident and wish to present it all at the end). It is sometimes difficult to differentiate fat from distension (which can be due to flatus, fluid, foetus, faeces or tumour).

Next, hold the hand and look for any nail changes and hand signs (e.g. clubbing, palmar erythema), palpate the radial pulse, look into the mouth for furring of the tongue and for dry mucous membranes, look into the eyes for jaundice or anaemia (pale conjunctiva) and swiftly feel the neck for any lymph nodes (including Virchow's node). On palpation of the abdomen (make sure your hands are warm) kneel down to the patient's

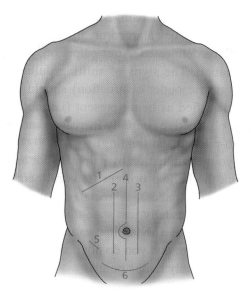

Figure 9.2. Abdominal incisions: (1) right subcostal or Kocher's incision, (2) right para-median, (3) left paramedian, (4) midline, (5) gridiron (Lanz), (6) Pfannenstiel. Note that many operations, including appendicectomy and cholecystectomy, are carried out laparascopically nowadays and the port-site scars may be small and difficult to see, or hidden within the umbilicus.

right, so that you are roughly level with them. The abdomen can be divided into theoretical regions as in Figure 9.1.

Starting at the furthest point from where the patient tells you the pain is, gently palpate in each of these regions. This gives you a quick idea of any obvious masses or tender areas and whether the abdomen is soft. You should begin to think of what anatomical structures are under this area. Always look up at the patient's face (for grimacing). Next you can palpate a little deeper to build up on the findings of gentle palpation. Note if there is any guarding, rigidity or rebound. Rebound tenderness (most painful when the examining hand is removed) is not a good test, as it often causes the patient unnecessary pain and can give equivocal results. Tenderness on percussion is a more accurate and kinder way of assessing the same thing. Examine the liver and spleen (starting in the right iliac fossa for both, with the patient breathing in each time you press in) and ballot the kidneys. In

10

BREAST SURGERY

Tom Lennard

EXAMINATION

Breast cancer is a common disease and a core topic which frequently comes up in exams. You need to be proficient in the examination of the breast which is best achieved by attending breast clinics and clerking in patients who are scheduled for surgery. Intimate examinations such as this can be difficult because it takes a lot of effort to make the anxious patient feel at ease. You may be even more nervous or embarrassed than the patient and you must always offer the patient a chaperone.

Inspection

Tell the patient what you are going to do and the order you would like to do it in so she knows what to expect. Ask the patient to sit on the side of the bed, exposing the upper half of her body. If the patient has found a lump ask her to point to it. With her arms relaxed at her side, observe for any obvious asymmetry or masses, skin dimpling, previous scars and inversion or eczema of the nipple. Then ask her to raise her arms straight above her head, which strains the ligaments of Astley Cooper and may bring to light a previously unnoticed skin dimple or inversion of the nipple caused by an underlying breast cancer. Now ask her to put her hands on her hips and push inwards. Check that the pectoralis major is contracted and ask her to relax and contract whilst observing the breast for dimples and inversion of the nipple.

Palpation

Now ask the patient to lie down with her arms by her side. Start with the normal breast first. Hold the patient's arm so that it is abducted to 90°, allowing the pectoral muscles to be relaxed as you take the weight of the arm. This will permit easy examination of the axilla and spreads the breast tissue over the chest wall.

The breast extends from the second rib to the inframammary fold. The breast is divided into five areas: the four quadrants and a central nipple area. Palpate each area using the flat surface of your fingers as a paddle and the chest wall as the counterplate against which you are pressing the tissue of the breast. This should enable palpation of any masses. Normal breast tissue varies between women and with the stage of the menstrual cycle, so by examining the patient's normal breast first, you will effectively have a control against which to compare the other side. Now examine the symptomatic breast.

If you find a lump, note its site, size (by measuring it with your ruler), shape, surface, edge, consistency and relation to surrounding structures (skin and underlying muscle). To assess if the lump is tethered to muscle, ask the patient to place her hands on her hips and push inwards. This will tense the pectoralis major muscle; if the lump is fixed to that, its mobility when you move it will decrease. If the patient complains of a discharge from the nipple, ask her to demonstrate it. Note the colour and viscosity of the fluid and whether it comes from one or more ducts. If discharge is elicited then place a glass slide onto it so a cytology smear can be obtained.

An essential part of breast examination is the assessment of the regional lymph node drainage areas, the axilla, the neck and the supraclavicular fossae. To examine the axilla, the pectoralis major and latissimus dorsi need to be relaxed, so take her arm, abduct it to 90° and insert your fingers into the axilla (be gentle). Note any palpable lymph nodes. This is a sensitive area of the body and you will need to be careful not to cause discomfort or tickle the patient. Complete your examination of the nodal area by palpating the neck and supraclavicular fossae. It is important to log the findings of your examination in your mind as you go along, so when you are palpating the lump you should be thinking or running through the checklist: what is the site, size, shape, etc. This helps you to remember to check all the necessary features and is easier than doing the examination and then trying to remember what you found, or even worse, realising that you missed out or forgot to assess, for example, the nodal basin or the size of the mass.

Tell the examiner your findings. For example: "This lady has a 3 cm hard lump in the upper outer quadrant of the right breast. It has a smooth surface and a well-defined edge. It is mobile and not attached to the skin or underlying muscle and is not tender. There are two nodes palpable in the right axilla. They are soft and mobile. There are no nodes palpable in the supraclavicular fossa. My differential diagnosis is either a cyst, fibroadenoma or possibly a breast cancer." The order in which you should give this differential depends on your clinical suspicion, which is influenced by the age of the patient and your findings.

BREAST CANCER

Breast cancer affects 1 in 10 women in the UK. The risk of developing breast cancer by the age of 50 is 1 in 50; by age 65, 1 in 17; and by age 85, 1 in 9. The incidence of breast cancer increases with age and is the commonest cause of cancer-related deaths in females aged less than 54 (Figure 10.1).

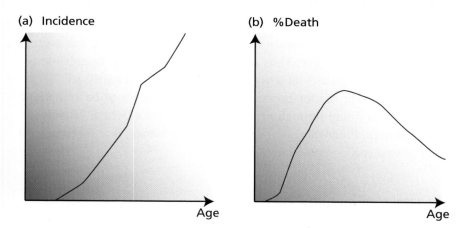

Figure 10.1.   (a) Incidence of breast cancer vs. age; (b) percentage of deaths attributable to breast cancer vs. age.

Risk Factors

There are multiple interrelated risk factors. Overall only 15% of women with breast cancer have an identifiable risk factor apart from age and gender which are of course the major factors. Male breast cancer does occur but is much rarer, accounting for about 1 per 500 breast cancers.

Family History

Around 4–10% of breast cancers are due to an inherited trait. Overall, if a first-degree relative has had breast cancer under the age of 40, or has had bilateral breast cancer, then a woman has double the normal risk. The inheritance pattern is usually an autosomal dominant trait with variable penetrance. In other words, you may inherit the gene from your father or mother, but your risk of getting breast cancer will not be 100%. The commonest breast cancer genes to have been identified are the BRCA1 and BRCA2 genes (on the long arms of chromosomes 17 and 13 respectively). BRCA1 affects 2% of Ashkenazi Jews. BRCA1, but not BRCA2, is commoner in patients with a family history of breast and ovarian cancer. Women with either of these genes have a 40–80% lifetime risk of developing breast cancer.

Exposure to Oestrogens

In general the longer a woman has periods and the later she has a pregnancy the greater the risk. Thus a late menarche, an early menopause (or ovariectomy), pregnancy at a young age and increased parity are associated with a lower risk of breast cancer. There appears to be something about a breast going through pregnancy and lactation which "stabilises" the epithelium. Pregnancy after the age of 35, however, is associated with an increased risk compared to nulliparity.

The Oral Contraceptive Pill (OCP)

Use of high-oestrogen-content (50 µg or more) oral contraceptives for greater than four years before the first pregnancy increases the risk of premenopausal breast cancer. Women who use the OCP for short periods to space pregnancies are at no increased risk.

Hormone Replacement Therapy (HRT)

Menopause occurs in women in the UK at a median age of 50 years. Women who have experienced early menopause for any reason can take HRT up to the age of 50 with no concerns as they would normally have had circulating hormones up to that timepoint anyway. In that context it is truly replacement therapy. HRT taken beyond the age of 55 years carries small increases in risk of breast cancer, typically 3–5 extra cancers per 1000 women over the following five years. The risk seems to return to the normal population risk after five years of stopping the HRT, i.e. the risk is not sustained for life but is transient. The Million Women Study has demonstrated that oestrogen-only HRT carries the smallest increase in risk, whereas with combined oestrogen-progesterone HRT the risk is greater. There is currently considerable doubt whether HRT should be prescribed to prevent osteoporosis or heart disease, but as a short-term bridge for women with bad menopausal symptoms it is a very effective treatment.

Previous Benign Breast Disease

Fibroadenomas and most types of benign breast disease are not a risk factor. Atypical epithelial hyperplasia on breast biopsy, particularly with a positive family history, does, however, increase the risk for breast cancer.

Other Factors

Breast cancer has a low incidence in Asia and Eastern Europe. Obesity increases the risk in postmenopausal women. The source of oestrogens in these women is the peripheral aromatisation of androgens produced by the adrenal glands. High socioeconomic status, a diet high in saturated fats and high alcohol intake are also linked with an increased risk of breast cancer. Smoking does not seem to be a risk factor.

(DCIS) may present just as a cluster of microcalcification. The X-rays from the right and left breasts should be juxtaposed on the viewing box to assess symmetry. Ask a radiologist to show you how it is done. Mammography misses about 7% of palpable breast cancers in women over 50 years, rising to about 20% in premenopausal women who have dense impenetrable breast tissue. Lobular carcinoma (around 10% of all breast cancers) is the classical type of breast cancer missed on mammography, and magnetic resonance imaging (MRI) may be more sensitive in sizing and assessing lobular cancers because of the lack of sensitivity of mammography with this subtype. Mammography remains the only proven screening tool for use in detecting breast cancer, and can be used to sample impalpable areas of concern (stereotactic biopsy).

Ultrasound

This is used in conjunction with mammography and can increase the accuracy of the radiological diagnosis of a lump. However, it does not usually "see" microcalcification, and is operator-dependent. It is not useful as a screening method for breast cancer but excellent for clarifying the nature of mammographic mass lesions and performing guided biopsies. Ultrasound is also used to assess axillary nodes.

Core Biopsy

If the FNA score is C1 or C3 and radiology and clinical examination is suspicious of breast cancer, then a core biopsy is performed. This allows a histological diagnosis to be made on the lump and discriminates between invasive and *in situ* cancer. The patient returns to the clinic after a few days for the result.

A bleb of local anaesthetic is injected into the skin overlying the lump, followed by deeper infiltration. The skin is then punctured with a scalpel blade and the core biopsy needle pushed into the lump. Most needles have an automatic firing mechanism or are attached to a "gun", resulting in a core of tissue being captured within the sheath of the needle. Core biopsy and FNA may be performed freehand if the lesion is palpable or guided using ultrasound and/or mammography with a stereotactic machine integrated with a digital mammography machine (Mammomat). Percutaneous removal of benign lesions of up to 1 cm or, where needed, larger biopsies of uncertain lesions can be achieved using guided vacuum-assisted biopsy devices.

Clinical Staging

Once the diagnosis of breast cancer has been confirmed by histology, then the patient is clinically staged. This is used to decide on the initial treatment options. Several staging or scoring systems exist, and although you don't need to learn any single system by heart, you do need to understand the principles. The TNM staging system is dependent on the size of the tumour and whether it has spread to the lymph nodes or more distant sites. This is outlined in Table 10.1.

Early breast cancer is clinical Stages I and II, whereas advanced breast cancer is Stage III and Stage IV. Clinical staging based on clinical findings is not accurate and therefore may need to be revised once further information, such as histology, becomes available.

Table 10.1. TNM Staging System

	Definition	Clinical stage equivalent
Tumour size		
T1	Tumour <2 cm	I
T2	Tumour 2–5 cm	I
T3	Tumour >5 cm	II/III
T4	Direct extension to skin or chest wall	III
Nodes		
N0	No palpable lymph nodes (LNs)	I
N1	Mobile LNs on same side	I/II
N2	Fixed LNs on same side	III
N3	Supraclavicular or infraclavicular LNs or arm lymphoedema	III
Metastases		
M0	No evidence of distant metastases	I/II/III
M1	Distant metastases present	IV

surrounding margin excised. While the patient is still on the operating table the excised specimen is X-rayed to ensure that the entire area of calcification has been removed. If mastectomy is performed then in certain circumstances immediate reconstruction can be done at the same time; however, if there are contraindications to immediate (e.g. significant comorbidity or possible need for postoperative radiotherapy) then delayed reconstruction may be more advisable. Not all women want reconstruction.

The surgeon should always perform the operation defined on the consent form and no more.

Treatment of the Axilla

The number of lymph nodes in the axilla is variable (up to 30). The presence of involved axillary lymph nodes is the single best predictor of survival from breast cancer. The cells of the primary breast cancer invade into the local lymphatics and the local blood vessels and the number of local lymph nodes containing tumour reflects the probability of widespread metastases. The aim of operating on the axilla is twofold: first, to prevent the uncontrollable growth of cancer when it is present, and second, to establish the prognosis (the risk of recurrence and death) of the patient.

To determine whether nodes contain tumour, the use of ultrasound preoperatively with guided FNA can help sort out the node-positive patients who need an axillary node dissection to remove the nodal basin. If the scan and or FNA are clear and suggest no nodal disease, then to minimise unnecessary axillary dissection and its attendant morbidity, sentinel node biopsy is performed. This requires the preoperative labelling of the sentinel node by radioisotope and blue dye injection into the skin of the breast just prior to operation. The surgeon uses the combined method of radioisotope and colour to track or see the relevant nodes and removes just them. If histology reveals a positive sentinel node, a second operation to clear the rest from the axilla is indicated.

In some centres imprint cytology of these nodes can be checked during the surgery, and if this identifies malignant cells, clearance of the nodal basin can be performed in the same sitting. This technique, however, is only 60% sensitive, meaning some patients will have negative imprint cytology only to find after full examination of all the nodes that they are node-positive after all. Axillary sampling (largely an obsolete operation now) involves removing the lower part of the axillary fat pad with its nodes. Axillary clearance involves removing the nodes either up to the axillary vein (level 1), medial border of the pectoralis minor (level 2) or border of the first rib (level 3) (Figure 10.2). The more extensive the node removal, the greater the risk of damage to the sensory nerves of the axilla (intercostobrachial nerves) and the development of lymphoedema of the breast, hand, forearm and/or arm.

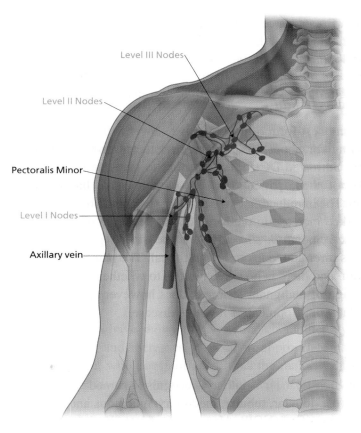

Level III Nodes

Level II Nodes

Pectoralis Minor

Level I Nodes

Axillary vein

Figure 10.2. The axillary lymph nodes.

and particularly those regimens containing anthracyclines are more effective than single-agent chemotherapy. Six cycles of cytotoxic chemotherapy given about once per month is the norm. Adjuvant endocrine therapy is not used if the primary breast cancer does not contain oestrogen receptors. The optimal duration of endocrine therapy is five years. The drugs used are oestrogen-receptor antagonists, such as tamoxifen, in premenopausal women and the aromatase inhibitor class of drugs, such as Arimidex, in postmenopausal women. In addition to their effects on the existing breast cancer, these agents both reduce the incidence of new or contralateral breast cancer by up to 50%.

Ovarian ablation by chemical means or oophorectomy also effectively reduces the risk of recurrence and death from breast cancer in premenopausal women, but is rarely used nowadays.

The combination of endocrine and cytotoxic therapy is more effective than chemotherapy alone or endocrine alone for patients with hormone-receptor-positive tumours. Menopausal-type symptoms (hot flushes, vaginal dryness, pruritus and loss of libido) are common with endocrine therapy.

The most common cytotoxic chemotherapy regime given at present is FEC (5-fluorouracil, epirubicin and cyclophosphamide) as six cycles over about six months. The side effects include exhaustion, nausea, vomiting, hair loss, suppression of the bone marrow and infertility. There are other drugs available for the treatment of breast cancer. These include the taxanes and Herceptin (a humanised monoclonal antibody which binds to the HER2/neu oncoprotein).

Discussions regarding adjuvant treatments are complicated and may require at least two meetings with the oncologist and breast care nurse. Guidelines and the deliberations of the breast MDT will inform the discussion.

Treatment of Advanced Breast Cancer

Advanced breast cancer includes locally advanced breast cancer (Stage III), metastatic breast cancer at presentation (Stage IV) and patients with recurrent breast cancer. The investigation and treatment of these three separate groups of patients are very similar and depend on understanding the spread of the disease. Like any cancer, spread takes place in the following ways:

- *Direct extension.* The cancer spreads to the muscle and chest wall, resulting in fixity, and to the skin, resulting in ulceration, which may bleed and become infected.
- *Via lymphatics.* It spreads via the lymphatics of the breast, leading to blockage of the lymphatics and oedema of the overlying skin, which becomes pitted by the adherence of the sweat ducts and hair follicles, leading to the appearance of *peau d'orange* and lymphoedema of the arm. Direct extension from involved axillary nodes may cause axillary vein thrombosis and infiltration of the brachial plexus.
- *Via blood.* It spreads especially to the bones (resulting in bone pain and hypercalcaemia), lungs (dyspnoea and pleural effusion) and liver (abdominal pain and compromised liver function).
- *Transcoelomic spread.* For example, pleural seeding leading to a malignant pleural effusion.

A bone scan, CAT scan of lungs and liver and full blood count and biochemistry will detect the majority of these potential problems.

It is essential to know the oestrogen receptor (ER) status of the tumour. A patient with a Stage III breast cancer and no evidence of metastases may be treated with endocrine therapy or cytotoxic chemotherapy prior to surgery. This so-called neoadjuvant therapy often results in shrinkage of the primary tumour, allowing surgical resection, which may be followed with more chemotherapy and radiotherapy. Local recurrence of a breast cancer previously treated by wide local excision may be suitable for mastectomy if there are no metastases. Unfortunately, however, what appears as local recurrence is often a sign of widespread metastatic disease.

Only 15% of patients in whom metastases are discovered will survive for five years; life expectancy (50% mortality) is 2–3 years. Treatment is therefore palliative. If the patient has no symptoms then there is a reasonable argument not to treat. Bone metastases are often painful and cause hypercalcaemia and pathological fractures. Hypercalcaemia is a medical emergency and is treated with hydration (intravenous saline), diuretics this muscle pocket. The nipple is reconstructed in a subsequent operation. The aim of reconstruction is to create symmetry so augmentation or reduction of the opposite breast may be necessary.

BENIGN BREAST DISEASE

Breast tissue naturally undergoes cyclical changes during the menstrual cycle. Under the influence of oestrogen and progesterone during the luteal phase, there is epithelial proliferation and increased vascularity. This can result in lumpy breast tissue which is tender and may be painful. Lumpy breast tissue may be focal and persistent. It forms the major differential diagnosis for breast cancer.

In most cases (>90%) triple assessment and review of the patient will define the diagnosis, but in the rare case of persistent lumpiness or C3 cytology, core biopsy or open operative biopsy may be necessary to rule out a diagnosis of breast cancer.

The histology of benign breast disease spans a spectrum which includes epithelial hyperplasia, sclerosing adenosis, apocrine metaplasia and fibroadenoma. It is only epithelial hyperplasia with pleomorphism of the cells and nuclei which is a risk factor for the development of breast cancer.

Benign discrete lumps in the breast (fibroadenomas) consist of overgrowth of the collagenous mesenchyme which surrounds each terminal lobuloalveolar unit (TLAU) and usually present before the age of 30; benign cystic disease of the breast usually presents in the 5–10 years prior to menopause when the terminal ducts undergo apoptosis and leave an isolated TLAU, which continues to produce fluid. Fat necrosis is an inflammatory response after an injury to the breast. Fibroadenomas can be treated conservatively or excised as a day case procedure. They occasionally grow to a great size (giant fibroadenomas). There are other rare conditions such as phylloides tumour, lymphoma, metastatic disease from other sites and chronic infections such as tuberculosis.

Breast Pain

Breast pain is either cyclical, occurring in the week prior to menses, or unrelated to the menstrual cycle. The former is common and usually lasts for

4–5 days, easing during or shortly after menses. Evening primrose oil may help but must be taken for at least two months. Non-cyclical breast pain is a completely different condition and is unexplained. Characteristically, women have pain in the breast and nipple associated with pain in the axilla and radiation down the arm. In about 15% of cases it is associated with back pain and examination reveals marked tenderness.

Tietze's syndrome is due to costochondritis and is not truly a breast problem. The classical sign is pain on pressing the costal cartilage. The treatment is non-steroidal anti-inflammatory drugs (NSAIDs).

Breast Infection

This most commonly affects women of childbearing age and can be divided into those related to lactation and those not related to lactation.

Lactational infection occurs during breastfeeding. It presents with pain, swelling and tenderness. The usual organism is *Staphylococcus aureus*, and antibiotics should be started (usually flucloxacillin). If an abscess develops then this can be treated by repeated aspiration and antibiotics so that the woman can continue breastfeeding. If the abscess persists then breastfeeding should be stopped by switching the baby to a bottle and the abscess treated surgically by incision and drainage.

Non-lactational infection can affect the periareolar region and is often called periductal mastitis. Complications from this condition are commoner in women who smoke. The major ducts under the areola become dilated (duct ectasia), there may be a lymphocytic infiltrate in the interstitial tissues and the major complication is rupture of one or more of the ducts. This results in the development of a periareolar collection of purulent fluid which is usually sterile. If the collection ruptures through the skin, a mammillary fistula is established. These are difficult to treat successfully. Excision of the whole major duct system may be necessary.

Discharge from the Nipple

Nipple discharges can be many colours (blood-stained discharges are the most sinister) and can come from either a single duct or multiple ducts. Physiological nipple discharge is common and can range in colour from white to green or black. Other non-malignant causes of discharge include a duct papilloma.

A duct papilloma may present with a blood-stained discharge from a single duct and the differential diagnosis includes an underlying carcinoma, which must therefore be excluded. A careful history should be taken and an examination performed. It is important to note whether a single duct or multiple ducts are involved. The secretion should be sent off for culture and cytology. Some form of imaging of the breast is necessary in order to exclude an underlying cancer. If all the tests are normal and the discharge is from multiple ducts, treatment is duct excision (known as Hadfield's procedure). This does not always completely stop the discharge since preserving the nipple inevitably leaves some ducts. If a single duct is involved then the affected duct can be removed by microdochectomy, a procedure in which a probe is passed into the affected duct, which is then excised and sent for histology.

11

LUMPS IN THE HEAD, NECK AND SKIN

Monica Hansrani

Lumps in the head, neck or skin appear frequently in clinical exams, mainly because the patients are usually well and present with good signs that allow examiners to gauge if a student has a structured approach to clinical assessment.

When you examine any lump you should think of the following list of features: site, size, shape, colour, contour (edge), consistency, compressibility (fluctuance), temperature, tenderness, tethering, transilluminance, pulsatility and spread (this means examining the regional lymph nodes). Although it's a long list, by the time finals come round you should have practised this many times. It can be easily remembered by the mnemonic "SSS, CCCC, TTTT and PS".

Your approach to a lump should be akin to a detective accumulating evidence (see Chapter 1) — assess the size and symmetry; scars; changes to the overlying skin such as colour changes (erythema, melanin deposition, vitiligo); changes in texture such as flakiness (psoriasis); oedema associated with inflammation or infection; the presence of telangiectasia and pearlescence (basal cell carcinoma or BCC). Does the lump move in relation to the overlying skin or the underlying structures (for example, the thyroid gland moves when swallowing)? Note the distribution of the lump or lumps as these may give a clue to the pathology (such as the presence of actinic keratoses and squamous cell carcinomas on sun-exposed areas, or BCCs on the nose etc.). Note the firmness of the lump. For example, a lipoma is usually soft, whereas a solid and irregular lump might suggest malignancy. The presence of

fluctuance suggests that the lump might contain fluid. As with a lump anywhere in the body you should take a full history of the lump (see p. 8). Think
of the anatomical structures underlying your examining fingers from the
components of the skin to glands, lymph nodes, blood vessels and bones.
This is not an exhaustive list; however, it gives you some idea of the effec-
tiveness of using a patient presenting with a lump as a test of students'
knowledge and diagnostic skills. Taking the time to describe the lump fully
often gives you time to think and work things out. However, it is easy to
make a meal of it!

Don't forget to look and feel inside the mouth. Examine the facial
nerve function when you suspect a parotid lump. Remember to examine
draining lymph node groups if there is a chance that a lump could be malignant or infective. Remember also that common things occur commonly
and that, as well as lumps specific to the head and neck (e.g. thyroid),
lumps in the head and neck could also be general lumps that could occur
anywhere on the body (e.g. sebaceous cysts, lipomas, lymphomas, neurofibromas and skin tumours).

Try to avoid terms such as "nobbly" and make sure you use appropriate
medical terminology such as "macule", "papule", "plaque", "erythema" —
but be sure you know what they mean!

LUMPS IN THE HEAD AND NECK

Triangles of the Neck

Conventionally, lumps in the neck are described in relation to certain
anatomically defined landmarks (Figure 11.1). Lumps in the neck anterior
to the anterior border of the sternocleidomastoid muscle are within the anterior triangle of the neck (its boundaries are the sternocleidomastoid, the
midline and the lower border of the mandible). Lumps posterior to the anterior border of the sternomastoid are within the posterior triangle of the neck
(its boundaries are the sternocleidomastoid, trapezius and the clavicle). The
base of the posterior triangle is more commonly referred to as the supraclavicular fossa. Lumps under the jaw are in the submandibular region.

Therefore, if you are shown a lump in the neck, decide which triangle
it fits into and you may almost have the diagnosis already. Remember that

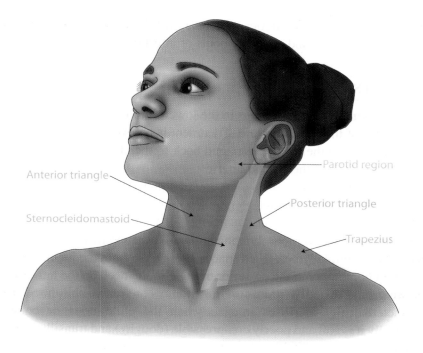

Figure 11.1. The triangles of the neck.

lymph nodes can occur in any of the areas (including the parotid) and can be multiple or single, while lumps in the midline (that are deep to the skin) are most likely to be of thyroid origin or thyroglossal cysts.

Branchial Cysts

Branchial cysts are congenital epithelial cysts believed to represent retained elements of the second branchial cleft which failed to disappear during embryological development. They are not apparent at birth but appear subsequently, usually in young adult life. A branchial cyst will usually be a swelling emerging from the anterior border of the sternomastoid muscle at the junction of its upper and middle thirds. They are bilateral in 2–3% of patients. Lined by squamous epithelium, they contain a so-called glary fluid containing cholesterol crystals and are often surrounded by lymphoid tissue. Surgical excision may be difficult due to the close proximity of the internal

and only then do a more general examination of the thyroid, including hands and eyes, if you think the lump is in the thyroid gland.

Here is a brief guide to the examination of a thyroid mass. First, inspect the neck from the front, looking for masses. If a mass is seen, ascertain if it moves up on swallowing. This is best done by asking the patient to take a mouthful of water. A glass of water next to the patient in an exam is often a clue that they are a thyroid patient. If there is no glass of water, always ask the examiners for one. Next, check that the trachea is central by placing a finger in the suprasternal notch and then feel the neck by standing behind the patient. Do not be afraid to ask the patient to move their chair forward if it is against a wall. Palpate the thyroid. If a lump is present, decide on its size and whether it is solitary, multiple or a diffuse enlargement of the whole gland. Again ask the patient to take a mouthful of water and hold it in the mouth. With your hands palpating the gland, ask them to swallow and see if the lump moves upwards. Now feel for cervical lymphadenopathy and other neck lumps. Then go around to the front again, look into the mouth for any lingual thyroid (at the back of the tongue) and percuss over the sternum for dullness (which may indicate retrosternal extension) and listen for a bruit (present in the thyrotoxic patient when the thyroid is very vascular). If you suspect thyroid disease, then the hands are inspected for temperature, tremor, pulse rate (tachycardia or atrial fibrillation). There are five eye signs that go with Graves' disease (exophthalmos, lid retraction, lid lag, ophthalmoplegia and chemosis).

If the thyroid feels normal, examine for lymphadenopathy or any other lumps. If you cannot feel any lumps and there are no skin lesions, then check the neck pulses; listen for bruits, and test sensation and neck movements.

If you are asked to examine the neck of a patient, it is perfectly reasonable to examine as described and then say something like this: "This patient has a 4 × 4 cm lump just to the left of the midline that moves upwards on swallowing. This is consistent with a lump in the left lobe of the thyroid gland. The lump is firm, with a smooth contour. I could not feel any other lumps or any associated lymphadenopathy. The trachea is central. There is no retrosternal extension detectable clinically and I could not hear a bruit on auscultation. I would now like to examine this patient for signs of thyroid disease." The examiner will then either tell you to go on or, more likely, ask you what you would look for.

Goitre

The word "goitre" means any swelling of the thyroid gland. The pathology books can make the causes of goitre sound very complicated, but from a clinical perspective the situation is more straightforward. First, ascertain whether the swelling appears to involve the whole thyroid gland or whether it is a swelling in just part of the thyroid gland. This can be attempted on clinical examination, but in practice nowadays most goitres will require an ultrasound scan to fully decide this. Ultrasound also provides the opportunity for fine-needle aspiration (FNA) cytology of a solid lesion or aspiration of a cyst.

Causes of Goitre

- Diffusely swollen thyroid
  - Graves' disease (thyrotoxicosis in a younger person)
  - Hashimoto's thyroiditis (an autoimmune condition)
  - Multinodular colloid goitre with nodules too small to feel
  - Iodine deficiency, puberty, pregnancy or ingestion of goitrogens (rare)
  - Rarely, de Quervain's thyroiditis (also called subacute thyroiditis — usually a self-limiting condition)

- Multiple nodules in the gland
  - Multinodular colloid goitre (the commonest thyroid swelling to be seen in exams)
  - Multiple cysts
  - Multiple adenomas

- Solitary nodule in the gland
  - Cyst
  - Tumour (benign or malignant, primary or secondary — which is rarely the case)
  - Dominant single nodule in multinodular goitre

Multinodular Colloid Goitre

This is thought likely to be an autoimmune condition. It is more common in middle-aged women and there may be a family history. The goitre may be asymptomatic; however, it may be a cosmetic worry to the patient or it may actually be causing symptoms, usually by pressure on adjacent structures, i.e. dysphagia (pressure on the oesophagus) and stridor (pressure on the trachea). In the longer term it may lose its capacity to function, resulting in hypothyroidism. If it is asymptomatic, no intervention is likely to be required other than reassurance and tests to exclude a carcinoma. If it is causing symptoms, then usually a thyroidectomy will be performed. For benign colloid goitre the choice lies between a subtotal or total thyroidectomy. In the former, a small amount of thyroid is preserved in relation to the superior thyroid artery to protect the parathyroid glands and recurrent laryngeal nerves and also to retain some thyroid tissue to produce thyroxine and prevent hypothyroidism.

Solitary Thyroid Nodules

Clinical examination and ultrasound can determine whether the goitre consists of a single nodule or multiple nodules. However, the mainstay of diagnosis is by FNA for cytology which can be carried out in outpatients. This can also be under ultrasound guidance if lumps are small or close to the carotid arteries. This is very good for making a diagnosis although it cannot differentiate between follicular adenomas and follicular carcinomas. As discussed earlier, multiple nodules are usually benign whereas solitary nodules may be malignant. Occasionally a radioisotope scan is performed if the thyroid function tests show hyperthyroidism, in order to look for a toxic nodule. A nodule is said to be cold if it fails to take up radioiodine. Such a cold nodule has a 10% chance of being malignant. Radioisotope scanning has less of a role than it used to have. Fine-needle aspiration (if necessary under ultrasound guidance) should be the first-line investigation of any thyroid lump. However, if the lump is clinically suspicious a hemithyroidectomy may be performed to get a histological diagnosis.

Thyroid Cysts

Such cysts may present as lumps or cause pressure symptoms. Local pain caused by bleeding into the cyst can be troublesome. The important thing is to rule out malignancy. An FNA may be all that is required to show this is a simple cyst. An ultrasound scan will help if the diagnosis is in doubt. Treatment is by aspiration, but the cyst may require excision if cytology dictates or if it recurs.

Thyroid Function Tests (TFTs)

Thyroxine (T4) is the hormone produced by the thyroid. It is converted to the active hormone triiodothyronine (T3). The thyroid-stimulating hormone, TSH, is produced by the pituitary and stimulates T4 production.

There is a negative feedback mechanism in action:

- T3 and T4 are low and TSH is high in hypothyroidism.
- T3 and T4 are high and TSH is low in hyperthyroidism.
- T3 and T4 are normal and TSH is low in patients on adequate doses of T4.

Before any patient with thyroid disease is operated on, it is essential to know the thyroid status by sending off TFTs. Hyperthyroid patients must be controlled preoperatively with antithyroid drugs (usually carbimazole), and beta-blockers may be used. Lack of control might cause a thyroid crisis.

Some surgeons insist on having the vocal cords checked preoperatively to document any abnormalities prior to surgery.

Primary Thyroid Tumours

It must be emphasised that solitary thyroid nodules are benign most of the time (90% benign, 10% malignant). Fine-needle aspiration cytology usually dictates management.

- *Adenomas.* These are benign and may be either functioning (causing hyperthyroidism and appearing as "hot" on a thyroid isotope scan) or nonfunctioning (appearing as "cold" on a thyroid isotope scan). Treatment is usually by hemithyroidectomy and removal of the isthmus.
- *Carcinomas*
  - *Papillary carcinoma* (70%). This occurs in younger patients. It has the best prognosis of thyroid cancers. It is often multifocal.

Spread to cervical lymph nodes occurs but may not alter the good prognosis. Treatment is usually by hemithyroidectomy for uncertain cytology. If initial cytology gives a confident report (described as AC5) then total thyroidectomy would be recommended. Following a hemithyroidectomy, if the lesion is bigger than 1 cm, a completion thyroidectomy would be done. Since the tumour is sensitive to iodine, the patient is usually given radioiodine to target the metastases after a total thyroidectomy. This is performed postoperatively, so that it does not get concentrated in the thyroid gland. In a patient treated by hemithyroidectomy alone, thyroxine must be given to suppress TSH levels to less than 0.1.

o *Follicular carcinoma* (25%). This is also found in young adults and is characterised by follicular appearance on histology. It has a good prognosis if appropriately treated, although prognosis is poorer in older patients. When it spreads, metastases are blood-borne. A hemithyroidectomy is usually performed. In 10% of these cases a carcinoma rather than an adenoma is confirmed. The patient then has a completion thyroidectomy unless the lesion is 1 cm in size or less. Since the tumour is sensitive to iodine the patient is usually given radioiodine to target the metastases after a total thyroidectomy (postoperatively, so that it does not get concentrated in the thyroid gland). As in the case for papillary carcinoma, if a hemithyroidectomy is performed, thyroxine would be given afterwards for TSH suppression.

o *Medullary cell carcinoma* (5%). This is a tumour derived from the calcitonin-producing C-cells. It is relatively rare and is part of the MEN I syndrome. Cytology would pick this tumour up preoperatively and diagnosis would be confirmed by calcitonin measurement. Treatment is by total thyroidectomy. It does not take up radioiodine.

o *Anaplastic carcinoma* (rare). This is a highly aggressive and locally invasive tumour and is seen in older patients. The history is of rapid increase in size over about six weeks. It is usually incurable, and treatment is usually palliative but may involve a tracheostomy and external beam radiotherapy.

○ *Lymphomas.* Lymphomas, both Hodgkin's and non-Hodgkin's, may arise within the thyroid gland. This is suspected in a big goitre that is rubbery and has recently enlarged. Diagnosis should be made by FNA and open biopsy may be needed to classify the lymphoma. Treatment is primarily with chemotherapy which will also treat involved lymph nodes. Surgical excision is less often needed. Lymphoma may also develop in a gland affected by Hashimoto's thyroiditis.

Complications of Thyroid Surgery

A relatively common topic in surgical finals relates to the complications of thyroid surgery. The following are the important facts you need to know:

- *Acute haemorrhage.* Bleeding into the neck after thyroidectomy can be a life-threatening complication, as it can cause acute airway obstruction. If you are called to a patient in whom this is occurring, first contact the on-call anaesthetist who may need to intubate the patient. The clips should be immediately removed but deeper sutures may need cutting before the haematoma can be evacuated. The patient should be taken to theatre for the wound to be explored and bleeding stopped. This occurs in less than 1 in 100 operations.
- *Damage to the recurrent laryngeal nerve.* The nerve runs close to the posterior aspect of the thyroid gland and is at risk during thyroidectomy unless it is specifically identified and preserved. Damage may occur at the point of insertion into the larynx or when tying the inferior thyroid artery. Damage to one recurrent laryngeal nerve causes hoarseness of the voice; damage to both causes airway obstruction requiring tracheostomy (because the neutral position of the vocal cord is in the midline).
- *Damage to the parathyroid glands.* This may be due to poor blood supply or inadvertent excision. This produces hypocalcaemia resulting in tetany. The two physical signs of hypocalcaemia often asked about are Chvostek's sign and Trousseau's sign. Chvostek's sign is when twitching of the facial muscles occurs on tapping over the facial nerve at the posterior aspect of the parotid gland. Trousseau's sign is when carpal spasm is produced by blowing up a blood pressure cuff on the upper arm.
- *Hypothyroidism.* This is due to lack of functioning thyroid tissue.

Thyroglossal Cysts

In embryological development the thyroid starts at the foramen caecum at the back of the tongue and descends to its final position passing close to the hyoid bone. Remnants can be left at any point along this line of descent, including a very rare lingual thyroid (i.e. thyroid tissue at the back of the tongue). Care needs to be taken before excision of a lingual thyroid, in case it is the patient's only functioning thyroid tissue. The classical features of a thyroglossal cyst are that it is in the midline of the neck, and rises upwards on protrusion of the tongue. Such cysts can become infected. Excision involves removal of the central portion of the hyoid bone and may require dissection as far as the back of the tongue. A thyroglossal fistula can also occur, again invariably in the midline, but is not actually congenital; it usually occurs following infection or inadequate surgical removal of a thyroglossal cyst.

Parathyroid Glands

The parathyroids only very rarely produce a palpable neck lump (in fact it is so rare that it should probably never be suggested in an exam). The management of hyperparathyroidism is, however, a common question. Most cases of hyperparathyroidism are discovered by finding an elevated calcium on routine investigation. Remember that the symptoms of hypercalcaemia are "bones, stones, psychic moans and abdominal groans" and that hyperparathyroidism can be any of the following:

- *Primary*, i.e. spontaneous (85% due to an adenoma of one gland, 15% due to diffuse hyperplasia of all four glands). In most adenomas parathormone-related protein (PTH-rP) is produced.
- *Secondary*, where hyperparathyroidism is secondary to a low serum calcium such as is found in chronic renal failure and malabsorption syndromes (the PTH is therefore high, with a low or normal serum calcium).
- *Tertiary*, where in long-standing secondary hyperparathyroidism the gland has become autonomous (high PTH and normal or high calcium).

The surgical treatment of hyperparathyroidism is exploration of the neck through an incision similar to that used for thyroidectomy and identification of all four parathyroids. If the cause is an adenoma, it is removed. If it is hyperplasia of all four glands, then all four glands are removed.

Salivary Glands

The salivary glands consist of the parotid, submandibular, sublingual and other minor salivary glands. The parotid region is that part of the face in front of the ear and below the zygomatic arch. The gland is delineated into superficial and deep portions by the branches of the facial nerve. Hence it is important clinically to recognise that a lump may be in the parotid gland as simple excision could result in a VII nerve palsy.

The operation to remove most superficial lesions of the parotid (superficial parotidectomy) involves making a long incision in front of the ear and down onto the neck, and identifying the facial nerve as it enters the parotid gland. The branches of the facial nerve are then followed forward and the superficial part of the parotid gland dissected off them. If a parotid lump is easily palpable when examined bimanually with a finger in the mouth, it may be in the deep portion of the gland and excision is then associated with a much higher risk of damaging the VII nerve. The facial nerve supplies the muscles of facial expression, so test the nerve by asking the patient to smile, show you their teeth and close their eyes. You must always document your findings.

Acute Parotitis

The parotid gland is surrounded by a tough fibrous capsule, and when it swells, as in acute parotitis, the stretching of the capsule causes severe pain. This condition may be due to viral infection (mumps, Coxsackie A and others) or bacterial infection. Bacterial infections usually arise because of obstruction of the duct, due to calculus, or because of reduced salivary flow, such as in the postoperative patient or sick dehydrated patient from other causes. This is why mouth care is so important in such patients. Acute bacterial parotitis may result in abscess formation. You are unlikely to see a patient with this in an exam.

the lesions. They are usually small, firm, smooth and not fixed to skin or deeper structures.

Sebaceous Cysts

These follow obstruction to the mouth of a sebaceous duct. They are common on the scalp and groins, but can occur anywhere except the soles and the palms (which do not have sebaceous glands). Typically they form a round, soft, fluctuant swelling attached to skin but not deeper structures. Look for a central punctum which usually clinches the diagnosis. Sebaceous cysts contain cheesy material which smells and may become infected. Less commonly, they may ulcerate or form a sebaceous horn. They are usually simply removed under local anaesthetic. A coalescence of infected cysts, classically on the back of diabetics, can form a carbuncle with multiple openings.

Hidradenitis Suppurativa

This presents as a cluster of abscesses most commonly affecting the skin of the axillae, groins, inframammary, inner thighs and buttocks. This represents an infection in the apocrine glands, epidermoid, pilonidal and sebaceous cysts, which can be very distressing and disabling to patients. Drainage provides relief, but patients are prone to scarring and sinus formation. Flare-ups may be triggered by stress, perspiration, heat, clothing friction and hormonal changes.

Benign Naevi (Pigmented Moles)

These are developmental anomalies consisting of immature melanocytes in unusual numbers and sites within the skin. They are common, with an average of 16 present on the skin surfaces of most Caucasians. They come in a wide variety of shapes and sizes and are categorised by site, colour, cell type and depth. Surgically, the main importance of benign naevi is in the differential diagnosis of malignant skin lesions, principally malignant melanoma. Patients with dysplastic naevus syndrome, where there are multiple naevi with irregular margins and pigmentation, have a significantly higher risk of developing malignant melanoma.

Papillomas

Papillomas arise from either squamous or basal layers of the skin. They include the following:

- *Infective warts.* These are due to viral infection.
- *Keratin horns.*
- *Basal cell (seborrhoeic or senile) warts.* These are extremely common benign tumours of aging skin. They classically present as brownish, warty nodules or plaques on the upper trunk, head or neck and may have variegated colours from fawn to black. Usually multiple, they are mostly asymptomatic, but can catch on clothing, become inflamed and occasionally bleed.
- *Pedunculated papillomas (skin tags).* These are of no medical significance but may need removing if they are catching on clothes or are a worry cosmetically.

Vascular Malformations

- *Campbell de Morgan spots (cherry angiomas).* These red, dome-shaped spots appear as patients grow older and are of no clinical significance. They need no treatment.
- *Port wine stains.* These can occur anywhere, but most commonly on the face and scalp. They have a deep red discolouration due to dilated blood vessels and may be associated with an underlying meningeal angiomatous malformation when present over the ophthalmic area (Sturge–Weber syndrome).
- *Strawberry naevi (capillary angiomas).* These are raised purplish nodules or plaques which usually present at birth, but may develop in the first few months of life. They usually flatten and resolve with puberty but are occasionally associated with sequestration of platelets and underlying dermal ischaemia.
- *Cavernous haemangiomas.* These are composed of large vascular spaces and usually present as soft, compressible, mauvish-blue swellings which may vary in size from day to day. These do not resolve spontaneously and can be treated with surgical excision or sclerosants.

- *Venous lakes*. These are uncommon benign bluish saccular dilatations of the lip in elderly patients.
- *Glomus tumours*. These often occur around the fingertips as characteristic painful benign cuboidal lesions.
- *Pyogenic granulomas*. These characteristically are rapidly developing red, domed papules with a glazed or eroded surface, commonly found around fingers or toes (although they occur anywhere on the body) and usually resolve spontaneously after weeks to months.

Malignant Lesions

Melanomas

The incidence of malignant melanoma is rising sharply. Exposure to ultraviolet (UV) radiation (especially sunburn as a child) is thought to be the major aetiological factor.

Melanomas are highly malignant tumours derived from melanocytes and need to be diagnosed and removed early if a cure is to follow. They currently account for 4% of all skin tumours, but cause the greatest number of skin-cancer-related deaths.

Fair or red-haired individuals have the highest risk. The commonest sites are the torso in males and the legs in females (pointing to sun exposure as a risk factor). Rare sites include the nail bed (acral lentiginous), the anorectal junction and the choroid in the eye. If you come across a patient in the exam with a glass eye and an enlarged liver, think melanoma!

Patients with moles should be educated to look for the warning signs of changes in a mole using the "ABCDE" criteria:

- Asymmetry — half the lesion does not match the other half
- Border irregularity
- Colour variegation
- Diameter — any change in diameter should be assessed, but in particular a diameter >6 mm
- Evolving — changes in a lesion over time (particularly in nodular or amelanocytic lesions)

Any mole which either grows or appears rapidly, changes shape or colour, itches, ulcerates or bleeds should be regarded as suspicious and removed. You should examine the regional lymph nodes.

The types include the following:

- *Superficial spreading melanomas* (about 80%). These grow slowly and metastasise late, and have a better prognosis.
- *Nodular melanomas.* These invade deeply and metastasise early and have a poorer prognosis.

Total excisional biopsy is the method of choice for diagnosis, although in some circumstances (for example in a huge lesion) a partial biopsy is necessary. Sentinel lymph node biopsy is used to aid in staging of the melanoma.

You need to be familiar with two staging systems used for melanomas. The Breslow thickness is the depth of the tumour in millimetres and is the most important histological determinant of prognosis. Clark's staging, which breaks down the depth into five anatomical levels (e.g. Stage I — confined to the epidermis; Stage V — penetrated into the subcutaneous fat), has also been used in the past.

However, the AJCC (American Joint Committee on Cancer) *Cancer Staging Manual* 2010[*] no longer uses these as they were found to demonstrate less statistical correlation to prognosis. In practice the two systems are combined together with the histological grade to give a more accurate stage.

Prognosis

The thickness of the primary tumour is the single most important prognostic factor for patients with no evidence of distant spread. As a rough guide, Table 11.1 lists the five-year survival rates based on the depth.

Tumours in the back, arms, neck and scalp (BANS) areas tend to do worse than tumours on the periphery. Women seem to survive longer than

---

[*] American Joint Committee on Cancer (2010). *Cancer Staging Manual*, 7th Edition. New York: Springer.

Table 11.1.   Five-Year Survival Rates

Thickness (mm)	Five-year survival (%)
<0.76	96–99
0.76–1.50	87–94
1.51–4.0	66–77
>4.0	<50

men, and this may be due in part to their having more tumours on the legs than men. Various histological types (such as those with increased mitoses) and those with satellite lesions (implying that the dermal lymphatics are involved) have a worse prognosis. Ulceration is a poor prognostic indicator.

The surgical margins for resection are still controversial but, as a rough guide, impalpable lesions (thought to be <1 mm) should have a 1 cm margin whereas thicker palpable lesions (>1.5 mm) should have a 2–3 cm clearance. Survival is independent of the width of excision, but local recurrence may not be. Dissection of the regional lymph nodes is again a controversial subject, but most surgeons would agree that this should only be performed if they are clinically palpable. Other modalities used include chemotherapy and isolated limb perfusion of antineoplastic drugs, although with limited success and prognosis is not greatly improved. Close follow-up of outpatients is important in order to detect recurrence early.

Basal Cell Carcinomas (BCCs)

Basal cell carcinomas are very common lesions and are often asked about in finals or seen as short cases. They are low-grade malignancies, rarely metastasising, but they can erode into bone or other adjacent structures if they are left to grow large enough. Exposure to sunlight is a risk factor but they do not occur until middle age or later. 90% are found on the face, usually above a line from the lobe of the ear to the corner of the mouth. Early lesions consist of a raised, pearly pink papule with fine telangiectasia over it. Later the lesion ulcerates and is often called a "rodent ulcer". Treatment is usually by surgical excision, although cryotherapy or radiotherapy is sometimes used.

Squamous Cell Carcinomas (SCCs)

Squamous cell carcinomas are less common than basal cell carcinomas, but once again exposure to sunlight is a risk factor. With these and BCCs a cumulative effect of UV light appears to be important, whereas with melanomas short periods of intense exposure (burns) appear to be responsible. SCCs are more malignant than BCCs and may arise in pre-existing lesions such as leg ulcers (where they are called Marjolin's ulcers). Metastasis is often to regional lymph nodes, which should always be examined. Treatment is by excision, with radiotherapy being used to treat recurrence or involved lymph nodes.

Bowen's Disease

Bowen's disease is an intraepidermal squamous carcinoma *in situ* and may progress to squamous cell carcinoma in 3–5%, a third of which metastasise. Controversy remains as to whether it is also associated with internal malignancies. It most commonly occurs in sun-exposed areas in Caucasians, but particularly the head and neck of men and the lower limbs and cheeks of women. It is characterised by single or multiple slowly growing well-defined brownish plaques, which are slightly raised and scaly. It may also occur on mucous membranes and is referred to as erythroplasia of Queyrat when it involves the glans penis. These lesions are usually treated with surgical excision with a 4 mm margin, but can be treated with topical antineoplastic drugs, radiotherapy or photodynamic therapy.

Kaposi's Sarcomas

These tumours are increasingly seen because of the association with HIV and immunosuppression in transplantation. They usually consist of nodules or plaques which may be red, purple, brown or black. They may be single or multiple, and though most commonly found on the skin, may also be found in the mouth, gastrointestinal and respiratory tracts. Their growth is variable in rate and a rapid rate of growth is associated with high mortality. Treatment is of the underlying cause. Surgery is not recommended due to recurrence at excision margins.

complete or incomplete (i.e. not surrounding all the contents), as is found in a sliding hernia.

- *Neck.* The neck of a hernia is the margin of the defect through which the hernia has emerged.
- *Reducible.* A hernia is reducible when its contents can return to the abdominal cavity either spontaneously or with manipulation.
- *Irreducible.* The hernia cannot be reduced despite pressure or manipulation.
- *Incarcerated.* This term is usually used to describe an irreducible hernia where the irreducibility is due to adhesions within the sac in the absence of obstruction or strangulation. However, to avoid confusion, it is best simply to refer to a hernia as being irreducible but not obstructed or strangulated, as others may not know what you mean by the term "incarcerated".
- *Obstructed.* The bowel within the hernia is obstructed. The patient may have the four cardinal signs of obstruction (pain, vomiting, distension and constipation).
- *Strangulated.* The blood supply to the contents of the hernia is occluded by pressure at the neck of the hernia. If the bowel is within the sac, the viability of the bowel is impaired. Usually the veins are occluded first and then further swelling leads to arterial occlusion, which precedes gangrene developing. If the hernia contains only omentum, then this too can strangulate, but in this case bowel obstruction does not occur.
- *Sliding hernia.* A sliding hernia is one which contains a partially extraperitoneal structure, such as the caecum on the right or the sigmoid colon on the left. Therefore, the sac does not completely surround all the contents of the hernia. The importance of this is that particular care must be taken when excising the sac, to avoid damaging the bowel.
- *Richter's hernia* (see Figure 12.1). This is where just part of the bowel wall is caught in the sac and may become strangulated. Because only part of the bowel wall is in the sac, the patient is not usually obstructed.
- *Herniotomy.* This term is used to describe the surgical procedure of ligation and excision of the hernia sac.
- *Herniorrhaphy.* This term is used for actual repair of the hernial defect.

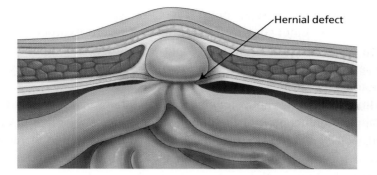
Hernial defect

Figure 12.1. Richter's hernia.

A common history of a groin hernia would be that the patient notices a lump in the groin that is reducible, and this may go on for years. Then, one day, the lump becomes irreducible, implying that it has become incarcerated. The patient may be well at this point. The lump may then become painful and the overlying skin reddened, implying strangulation (there may or may not be symptoms of obstruction, depending on whether there is bowel within it). At this point it becomes a surgical emergency and the patient requires an urgent operation to relieve the ischaemia and repair the hernia. If bowel has been irreversibly damaged it will need resection.

CLASSIFICATION OF HERNIAS

Hernias require a defect in the wall of their normal cavity for their formation. This defect may be congenital or acquired.

Congenital

The commonest types of congenital hernias are inguinal and umbilical hernias appearing in childhood.

Infantile inguinal hernias are usually seen in males (nine times more often). In males, when the testes develop and descend *in utero* they pass down through the abdominal wall into the scrotum, forming what will subsequently develop into the inguinal canal. As this happens, a finger-like projection of peritoneum, called the processus vaginalis, is carried down with the testicle.

This usually obliterates, but if it remains patent, fluid or abdominal contents may enter down it, forming either a hydrocoele (fluid around the testicle) or a hernia (containing bowel or omentum). The treatment is simple operative ligation of the processus vaginalis, i.e. a herniotomy.

Umbilical hernias are commonly seen in infants and represent failure of complete obliteration of the umbilical opening. They often disappear spontaneously and rarely strangulate. Surgical repair should therefore be reserved for those which persist after the age of 3–4 and those with a defect greater than 1 cm in size.

Acquired

To acquire an abdominal wall hernia, a weakness of the abdominal wall has to be present. The following may be predisposing factors:

- Chronic cough
- Chronic constipation (and straining to pass faeces)
- Straining to void urine (prostatism)
- Severe muscular effort (heavy lifting)
- Obesity
- Weakening with age
- Surgery

GROIN HERNIAS

Groin hernias are the commonest type of hernia encountered in exams, and indeed they account for about 75% of all hernias. They may be either femoral or inguinal. Inguinal hernias are further divided into direct and indirect hernias. Inguinal hernias are proportionally more common in males than in females, and femoral hernias are proportionally more common in females than in males (possibly because of a wider pelvis and hence wider femoral canal). In both sexes, however, inguinal hernias are more common than femoral hernias in absolute numbers. Read the last sentence again, as it is an important point that we don't want you to miss.

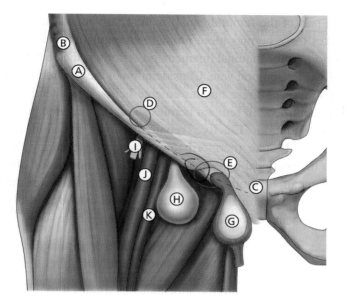

Figure 12.2. Anatomy of the groin: (A) inguinal ligament inserting into pubic tubercle, (B) anterior superior iliac spine (ASIS), (C) symphysis pubis, (D) deep inguinal ring, (E) superficial inguinal ring, (F) external oblique aponeurosis, (G) indirect inguinal hernia, (H) femoral hernia, (I) femoral nerve (outside femoral sheath), (J) femoral artery, (K) femoral vein.

Hernias may present in three ways:

- As a lump (which may come and go; classically the lump would appear on straining or lifting and disappear on lying down or when pressed on by the patient)
- With pain in the groin
- Because of a complication (obstruction or strangulation)

To understand groin hernias properly, some basic anatomical knowledge is required (Figure 12.2).

Femoral Hernias

Femoral hernias emerge through the femoral canal, which normally contains only fat and lymph nodes. The medial border of the femoral ring (the upper

the pubic tubercle). This point is slightly lateral to the midinguinal point which is the site of the femoral artery (midway between the anterior superior iliac spine and the pubic symphysis). However, most anatomy textbooks suggest that the deep inguinal ring is directly above the midinguinal point (i.e. above the femoral pulse), in which case the midpoint of the inguinal ligament becomes redundant as a landmark!

Here is a summary of how to examine a lump in the groin. For description purposes we shall refer to a male patient.

Introduce yourself and ask the patient if he minds your examining him.

Expose the abdomen, groins and legs. Ask the patient to stand, and inspect for any obvious lumps or scars and comment on your findings. If the patient is already lying down it is perfectly reasonable to perform the examination in this position; however, you must stand him up at the end of the examination, or you may miss small hernias, saphena varices and varicocoeles.

Examine the genitalia and both groins. If you can see an obvious lump, feel it gently and ascertain the features of the lump. Ask the patient to cough and feel for a cough impulse, listen over it for bowel sounds and ask him if he is able to reduce it. Once it is reduced, find the pubic tubercle and place your index finger on it. Ask the patient to turn his head away from you and then cough (so he doesn't cough on you!) and observe where the lump appears from in relation to your finger. An inguinal hernia will come out from the inguinal canal above and medial to your finger, whereas a femoral hernia will protrude below and lateral.

If you think this is an inguinal hernia, then state, for example, "The patient has a 5 cm smooth lump in his right groin. I think this is an inguinal hernia, because I cannot get above it, it is reducible, exhibits a cough reflex and protrudes above and medial to the pubic tubercle." The examiner might then ask you to tell if it is direct or indirect.

If a scrotal swelling is present, determine if it has an upper border, remembering that you cannot get above a hernia. Therefore, a lump with no upper border is likely to be an inguinoscrotal hernia. If you can get above it, then it is likely to be either a cord or a testicular lump. Ask yourself two questions: Is it separate from the testis and does it transilluminate? Do not forget to feel the epididymis and the skin of the scrotum as well (see Figure 14.1, p. 270).

Differential Diagnosis of a Lump in the Groin

Occasionally a lump in the groin will be something other than a hernia. The list of differential diagnoses includes the following:

- Inguinal lymph nodes (often multiple and usually below the inguinal ligament)
- Saphena varix, a dilated varicose vein at the sapheno-femoral junction (disappears on lying flat, and there may be other varicosities in the legs)
- Femoral artery aneurysm (pulsatile)
- Encysted hydrocoele of the cord (can get above it)
- Lipoma of the cord
- An incompletely descended testicle (absence of the testicle on that side)

Remember you cannot get above a hernia (this is a key point) and these other lumps will also not usually exhibit the classical features of hernia, which are as follows:

- Cough impulse
- Reducibility
- Bowel sounds heard over the hernia

Although a single enlarged femoral node can sometimes be difficult to distinguish from a strangulated femoral hernia containing omentum, such cases will rarely be seen in exams. Usually, if care is taken to examine the patient lying down and standing, the diagnosis will become obvious. Remember also to carefully examine both groins (as hernias are often bilateral) and the scrotum as there may be associated epididymal cysts or hydrocoeles to find.

OTHER TYPES OF HERNIA

Incisional Hernias

These can be simply defined as hernias which arise through a previously made incision. They are often broad-necked and, therefore, have a low risk of strangulation. Factors leading to the development of an incisional hernia include obesity, old age, chronic cough or straining due to constipation or prostatism (i.e. things which increase intra-abdominal pressure), post-operative wound infection or haematoma and poor surgical technique when the wound is closed. In high-risk patients, even large incisional hernias are often managed conservatively with an abdominal elastic support corset. Repair may be difficult and require the insertion of a nylon mesh to allow closure of the defect without tension. Again this can be done by either open or laparoscopic techniques.

Umbilical Hernias

In adults the hernia usually emerges adjacent to the umbilicus (unlike the congenital type) and is usually called "paraumbilical". Risk factors include the following:

- Cirrhosis/ascites
- Obesity
- Chronic cough
- Multiple pregnancies

Richter's Hernias

A Richter's hernia is where only part of the circumference of the bowel is within the sac. It is most often seen with femoral hernias. This is the only type of hernia which can strangulate without obstructing (other than a hernia which contains only the omentum). Although rather unusual in practice, it seems remarkably common in exam questions, which is why you need to know about it (see Figure 12.1).

Epigastric Hernia

This type of hernia arises in the midline through the linea alba. It is usually small and often difficult to feel, especially in overweight patients. It rarely contains bowel but often has extraperitoneal fat. It can cause symptoms out of proportion to its size, however, and patients often undergo unnecessary investigations for other causes of upper abdominal pain before the correct diagnosis is eventually made.

Spigelian Hernias

Again this type of hernia is very rare but common in exam questions. It is a hernia which occurs into the posterior rectus sheath at the point where the posterior sheath becomes deficient (i.e. at the arcuate line of Douglas).

Obturator Hernias

An obturator hernia occurs into the obturator foramen and does not usually produce a palpable lump. It is most commonly seen in thin elderly women, and pressure on the obturator nerve gives rise to pain felt on the inner aspect of the thigh. It is usually diagnosed only when obstruction has occurred, often not being suspected prior to laparotomy. The typical presentation would be a thin old lady with distension, vomiting, colicky abdominal pain, absolute constipation and pain in the inner thigh.

13

VASCULAR DISEASE

Gerry Stansby

INTRODUCTION

Vascular patients constitute a significant number of the cases seen in surgical finals. Most cases will be covered within the categories of arterial disease or venous disease, and most patients with venous disease will have varicose veins or venous leg ulcers. Questions about deep venous thrombosis (DVT) and pulmonary embolism (PE) are usually considered part of general medicine. The exception relates to prophylaxis against DVT for surgical patients — is a very common and topical question. Questions relating to cardiac surgery are not usually considered fair game for surgical finals except in relation to cardiology, which again comes under general medicine.

Unfortunately, many students are not given the opportunity to work in a vascular surgery unit and they often find this a confusing area when it comes to preparation for finals. As vascular surgery is a fairly specialised area, students will not be expected to know anything about the minutiae of the specialty. What is required, however, is a good knowledge of the principles of the following areas:

- How to examine the vascular system — arterial and venous
- Management of the acutely ischaemic leg
- Management of the chronically ischaemic leg/claudication
- Management of aneurysms
- Management of carotid artery stenosis

- Identification and treatment of risk factors such as smoking, diabetes and hyperlipidaemia

ARTERIAL DISEASE

Examination of the Peripheral Arterial System

Examination of the peripheral arterial system should be included as part of a full cardiovascular examination and as part of a full examination of a patient in the long case section of finals. However, it may be helpful to detail how one would carry out an examination restricted to the peripheral arterial system. First of all, one would inspect the patient for signs of peripheral arterial disease, such as ulcers, gangrenous toes, previous amputations, peripheral cyanosis and bypass surgery scars. In order to do this the patient must be adequately exposed. Do not forget to look for abnormal pulsations that might be caused by an abdominal aortic aneurysm. The examination then proceeds with inspection of the hands and feeling of the radial pulses. These should be felt individually on both sides and the two sides then compared. Look for nicotine staining. Likewise, the brachial pulses should then be felt and compared. The brachial pulse is best palpated just above the elbow crease on the medial aspect of the upper arm. A surprising number of patients have radial pulses which are difficult to feel, whereas the brachial pulse is usually easily palpable unless there is an arterial occlusion higher up. If there is doubt about the pulses being present or being equal, then you should suggest taking the blood pressure in each arm in order to get a more objective confirmation of this. There should not be more than 15 mm of mercury difference between the blood pressure in the arms unless there is a vascular problem. Such a difference will usually be due to disease in the aortic arch or subclavian vessels — rarely is it due to coarctation of the aorta.

The next part of the peripheral arterial examination is checking of the carotid pulses. Remember that the common carotid, which divides into the internal and the external carotid, is within the carotid sheath which lies under the anterior edge of the sternocleidomastoid muscle. The best way to feel the carotid pulse is with the patient's head resting on one pillow; ask them to look in the opposite direction, and then feel under the sternocleidomastoid. It is then important to listen for a bruit over the carotid. The best way to do this is to ask the patient to take a breath and then hold it whilst you listen with the diaphragm of the stethoscope. If you listen whilst they are breathing, you will find it difficult to hear soft bruits because of the noise made by the air moving in and out of the trachea. The process is then repeated for the carotid on the other side of the neck. Do not palpate the two carotids at the same time, as some patients may faint if that is done. If you are examining the cardiovascular system in general, then it would be appropriate at this point to move on to examination of the heart.

First of all, look for pulsation which might be caused by an aortic aneurysm, and then palpate for such an aneurysm. Then the abdomen should be auscultated for bruits. Remember that a bruit heard in the upper abdomen may be due to renal artery stenosis. Remember also that the bifurcation of the aorta is at the level of the umbilicus and so aortic aneurysms are usually felt in the upper abdomen.

The next stage of the arterial examination is to check the pulses in the groins and legs. The femoral pulse should be palpated on both sides and one side compared with the other. In coarctation of the aorta there may be radiofemoral delay. This is manifested by feeling the radial and femoral pulses simultaneously and feeling that the femoral pulse wave is occurring fractionally after the radial pulse. Coarctation of the aorta is, however, very uncommon. Such patients are usually young and often present with severe hypertension, so do not be tempted to overdiagnose this condition.

After palpation of the femoral artery, noting also whether it is of normal calibre or aneurysmal, auscultation of the femoral artery should be carried out to listen for bruits.

The next thing to do is to feel for the popliteal arteries. This should be done routinely, as otherwise one may miss a popliteal aneurysm. It is, however, often very difficult to feel the popliteal arteries in many patients, especially if they are overweight. Indeed, it is said that if one feels the popliteal pulse very easily, one should suspect immediately that there is a popliteal aneurysm present. There is no shame therefore for any student who says they cannot feel the popliteal arteries, but it is important that you do know how to examine them properly. The best way to proceed is as follows.

floor in order to gain some relief. The reasons the pain occurs at night are that we lose the effect of gravity helping to supply blood to the feet, the cardiac output drops when we are asleep, and the warmth of the bedclothes causes vasodilation in the skin, diverting the blood from the soft tissues.

Patients who have severe arterial disease sufficient to give them rest pain are usually classified as having critical ischaemia. Critical ischaemia can be loosely defined as ischaemia which is severe enough to threaten the loss of the limb or part of the limb. It can also be defined with the help of the ankle brachial pressure index.

Basically this involves taking the blood pressure in the foot, using a blood pressure cuff on the calf and a Doppler probe in order to pick up the foot pulse signal in either the posterior tibial or the dorsalis pedis pulse. The cuff is blown up until the signal disappears, and this is taken as the systolic pressure in the foot. This systolic pressure is then taken in a similar way in the arm, and the ratio of the two is calculated. The normal ABPI is 1 or slightly greater than 1. In claudication it is usually 0.5–0.9. Below 0.5 the patient may start to suffer from rest pain or, if more severe, necrosis or gangrene of the toes. Occasionally a claudicant may have a normal ABPI at rest, but this will be found to drop on exercise when an increased blood requirement to the muscles is limited by the stenosis.

Currently, most vascular surgeons would agree that patients with mild claudication are best managed conservatively, with the main advice being "Stop smoking and keep walking". In addition, medical problems such as anaemia, hypertension, hyperlipidaemia, diabetes and heart failure should be corrected. Overweight patients should be advised to lose weight. All patients should be on an antiplatelet agent (e.g. aspirin) and a statin. Risk factor management will be similar to that for cardiac patients. For more severe claudication or where there is thought to be a high chance of an iliac artery lesion, an angiogram should be arranged to see if there is an angioplastiable lesion.

Treatment of patients with chronic arterial disease may be carried out either by radiological intervention, i.e. balloon angioplasty, or by surgery. Balloon angioplasty consists of passing a special catheter into the narrowed area of the artery. The balloon on the end of the catheter can then be blown up to a high pressure to stretch open the narrowing. Sometimes stents are also used as in the coronary arteries. Angioplasty is a good technique in that it does not involve an anaesthetic and can be done with relatively little risk to the patient. It is particularly useful for narrowings or short occlusions of the iliac arteries but is less good for disease below the inguinal ligament.

Usually, only when there is either critical ischaemia or severe claudication which is making the patient's life intolerable should surgery be considered. In general terms there are only a small number of vascular surgical procedures which are commonly carried out and specific details will not be required for surgical finals. Occlusion in the aorta or iliac artery is usually treated by an aortabifemoral bypass graft, in which an artificial graft, usually made of Dacron®, is taken from the aorta above the blockage down to the femoral arteries in the groin. In patients who are considered too unwell to undergo this fairly major procedure, the femoral arteries can be revascularised by taking a graft from the axillary arteries just beneath the clavicle and running this down the sides of the thorax and abdomen under the skin into the groin arteries. In a patient with one good femoral pulse but a blocked iliac artery on the opposite side, a similar result can be achieved by taking a graft from the good common femoral artery across the subcutaneous tissue suprapubically into the ischaemic leg. This is called a crossover graft.

For blockages further down the leg, either a femoropopliteal or a femorodistal procedure may be performed ("distal" in this context means "distal to the popliteal artery", i.e. to one of the three tibial vessels — the posterior tibial, anterior tibial and common peroneal). The preferred choice of graft for these bypasses is usually the long saphenous vein, which may be either used with its valves destroyed by a special valve-cutting instrument or reversed so that the valves do not interfere with blood flow. Only if a suitable vein is not available do vascular surgeons resort to using an artificial graft material for grafts below the inguinal ligament. The commonest artificial material used below the inguinal ligament is polytetrafluoroethylene (PTFE).

Aneurysms

The word "aneurysm" comes from the Greek word for "widening" and is usually applied to abnormal widening of the arteries. Aneurysms can be found at various sites within the arterial circulation (e.g. aortic, femoral which have the purpose of preventing the pressure within the deep system from entering the superficial system. If these valves go wrong (i.e. become incompetent), then the superficial veins dilate up and appear as varicose veins. The common sites where this may occur in the lower limb are first at the long saphenous femoral vein junction in the groin (this is the commonest site), second at the short saphenous popliteal vein junction in the popliteal fossa behind the knee, and third from so-called perforating veins (veins which pass directly from superficial to deep) which become incompetent (Figure 13.3). Calf perforating veins are usually found on the medial side of the calf. Typically there are three: one just above the medial malleolus, one a hand's breadth higher and one a hand's breadth higher than that. In addition, some patients have a perforator in their medial thigh which is usually connected to the long saphenous vein. The position of perforators may, however, vary.

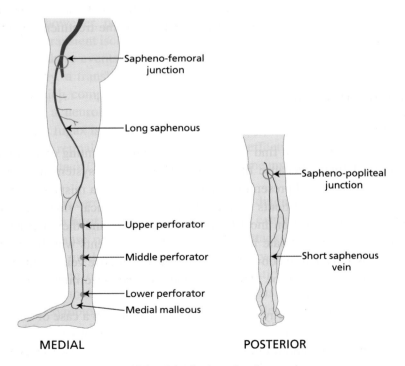

MEDIAL   POSTERIOR

Figure 13.3.   Distribution of varicose veins.

When one is assessing a patient with varicose veins, it is therefore important to try to categorise the varicose veins into three groups:

- Long saphenous veins
- Short saphenous veins
- Veins arising from calf perforators

In addition, the patient may have disease of the deep veins which may either be obstructed or incompetent, or may have a leg ulcer.

Points in the History

It is important to ascertain what it is about the varicose veins that troubles the patients. They may just be worried about them from a cosmetic point of view. Alternatively, they may be getting aching pains which are usually worse after a period of standing. Some patients find that they get swelling of the ankles, again most often after a period of standing. Varicose veins do sometimes cause cramps and other non-specific pains in the leg, but one must always be on the lookout for other pathology which might be causing the pain, as many patients will immediately ascribe pain from any cause (arthritis of the knee, for example) to their obvious and visible varicose veins.

Other points in the history which are usually taken include asking for a family history of varicose veins, any previous medical history suggestive of deep venous thrombosis or pulmonary embolism and, most important, whether the patient, who is usually a young woman, is on the oestrogen-containing oral contraceptive pill as this is something that really should be stopped 4–6 weeks before surgery because of the risk of DVT. Most varicose veins in women seem to worsen after pregnancy, and it is also a good idea to enquire about the number of past pregnancies and whether the woman wishes to have further pregnancies in the future.

Points on Examination

Never forget that occasionally abdominal or pelvic masses (including pregnancy) or malignancies can present as varicose veins due to pressure on the inferior vena cava or iliac veins. A full examination of the abdomen should therefore be part of examining a patient for varicose veins. In an OSCE you may not be expected to do this by the examiner (because of a lack of time), but you should make a point of saying, "I would now wish to do a full abdominal examination."

Always examine the arterial pulses in the legs as well. This is especially important in patients who have a leg ulcer. Varicose veins are usually best seen with the patient standing up. The legs should be exposed from the groin to the toe. As with all clinical examinations, the inspection should come first. You should particularly be looking for the presence of any signs of current or past leg ulceration. In patients who have had long-standing varicose veins and venous hypertension, you may see the changes of skin pigmentation (the skin is brown in colour, due to haemosiderin deposits) or lipodermatosclerosis (there is atrophy and loss of elasticity of the skin and subcutaneous tissues). Because most patients with such significant skin changes will have calf perforator disease, and because the calf perforators are found on the medial side of the calf above the medial malleolus, these changes are usually most prominent in the medial lower calf.

In addition, you should inspect the veins to try to make some preliminary judgement as to whether it seems they are likely to be arising from the long saphenous, short saphenous or perforating system. Remember that the long saphenous vein runs from the groin down the medial aspect of the thigh and calf. The veins below the knee which arise from it will therefore be mostly situated on the medial side of the calf, and in a thinner patient you may see a dilated varicose long saphenous vein running up the thigh. The short saphenous vein arises from the popliteal vein at a variable level within the popliteal fossa and then runs down the lateral side of the calf. By just looking at the legs with the patient standing, you may be able to make a good guess as to which of these two patterns the veins fall within. Calf perforating veins which are incompetent may produce very few varicosities but, as mentioned earlier, they will often be associated with significant skin changes like pigmentation and lipodermatosclerosis. Therefore, one can usually make a preliminary (educated) guess as to which of the three categories the veins fall into just on inspection.

Next comes palpation. Patients with a prominent saphena varix at the sapheno-femoral junction may actually have a lump visible in the groin, and this will need to be palpated to make sure it is not due to a lymph node or hernia. Otherwise, the mainstay of palpation is the tap test, whereby the veins are tapped down on the calf. Palpation over the saphenous vein in the thigh will reveal a transmitted thrill if the veins are in continuity and vice versa. It is also at the stage of palpation that one should quickly check the femoral, foot and popliteal pulses. Sometimes you may be asked about the so-called tourniquet test, or Trendelenburg test. Perhaps it is this which confuses more medical students than any other aspect of varicose vein examination.

It is now rarely done in vascular surgery clinics as the best form of assessment is with Doppler or ultrasound scanning. The principle of the test is that it is possible to compress the superficial veins by a tourniquet applied around the leg. The best way to describe the test in finals is elevation of the leg before applying a tourniquet as high on the thigh as possible.

The patient is then asked to stand and the veins are inspected to see if they refill rapidly. Remember that all varicose veins will refill slowly as blood passes through the arterial circulation, through the capillary bed and back into the venous system. What one is looking for is a rapid refilling within a few seconds, indicating that the tourniquet has not prevented the superficial reflux. For example, if there is sapheno-femoral junction reflux causing varicose veins, a high thigh tourniquet will prevent this rapidly refilling as the patient stands. If, however, there is short saphenous or calf perforator incompetence, the veins will fill rapidly despite a high thigh tourniquet. If the veins are controlled by the tourniquet in the thigh, then they are long saphenous veins due to sapheno-femoral reflux. If they are not controlled, the next manoeuvre should be to position the tourniquet just below the knee and repeat the test. If the veins are now prevented from refilling rapidly, then there is either sapheno-popliteal reflux or, very occasionally, a thigh perforator that is incompetent. If the veins continue to fill rapidly despite this tourniquet just below the knee, there is almost certainly calf perforator incompetence.

In reality, most vascular surgeons will want a duplex scan of the veins carried out before operating nowadays.

Varicose vein surgery is indicated for significant symptoms, skin changes or ulceration. Cosmetic treatments are not usually justified on the venous valve incompetence is present (usually following previous deep venous thrombosis), there is currently no good surgical procedure to improve deep venous function for most patients. For such patients the mainstay of treatment is to try to get the ulcer healed using the methods mentioned earlier and then to maintain healing by fitting a good-quality elastic graduated compression stocking. Patients who have their ulcers successfully healed should be encouraged to wear such stockings on a lifelong basis.

DEEP VENOUS THROMBOSIS (DVT) AND PULMONARY EMBOLISM (PE)

Management of deep venous thrombosis and pulmonary embolism is usually considered part of the medical finals. However, PE is the commonest preventable cause of death in surgical patients, and it is appropriate to be asked about it in surgical exams, especially in relation to prophylaxis. All hospital admissions should be assessed for DVT risk and prophylaxis given when the risk is elevated. Usually this means low-molecular-weight heparin and compression stockings, although newer oral anticoagulants are now in regular use, especially in orthopaedic patients. Not all DVTs are obvious clinically, although as the thrombosis progresses the leg may swell and become painful. At a later stage the leg may be extremely swollen, with impairment of skin circulation (phlegmasia caerulea dolens or phlegmasia alba dolens), and occasionally this may lead to venous gangrene. Pulmonary embolism may present in different ways. Massive pulmonary embolism will produce cardiorespiratory arrest and may initially be misdiagnosed as a primary cardiac problem.

A pulmonary embolism should always be suspected in a patient suffering a collapse or cardiac arrest within the first two weeks of a surgical procedure. Less major degrees of pulmonary embolisation may produce lesser degrees of collapse, or perhaps dyspnoea or pleuritic chest pain.

The treatment of DVT is anticoagulation, usually with heparin at first, followed by warfarin. Nowadays the majority of patients can be managed as outpatients with once-a-day injections of low-molecular-weight heparin whilst awaiting adequate warfarinisation. If a patient continues to have PEs despite adequate anticoagulation, then they should be considered for insertion of an inferior vena cava (IVC) filter.

Prophylaxis Against DVT in Surgical Patients

Patients having anything other than minor surgery should have prophylaxis against DVT. This is particularly so if they have any risk factors, such as older age, obesity, cigarette smoking, the contraceptive pill or a previous history of DVT or PE. The commonest type of prophylaxis employed is subcutaneous low-molecular-weight heparin. It is also common practice to use thromboembolic deterrent (TED) stockings, and many units have intermittent pneumatic compression devices which work by blowing up a series of cuffs on the leg and keeping the venous pump flowing even when the patient is immobile or in theatre.

LYMPHOEDEMA

This is an abnormal collection of interstitial lymph fluid either due to a congenital absence of the lymphatics (primary) or secondary to blockage of the lymphatics.

Primary lymphoedema can be present at birth (congenital lymphoedema), but more often it presents in the teens as lymphoedema praecox (Milroy's syndrome). This usually affects young females who present with progressive swelling (non-pitting) of one or both legs. Less often, it can present late at around the age of 30–40 and is then called lymphoedema tarda ("tarda" is Latin for "late").

Secondary lymphoedema can be caused by anything that damages or obstructs the lymphatics. The mnemonic "FIIT" is helpful for remembering the causes:

- Fibrosis, e.g. following radiotherapy
- Infiltration, e.g. by tumour, especially prostatic in men and lymphoma in women (in certain parts of the world, infestation with filariasis is a common cause of lymphoedema)
- Infection, e.g. tuberculosis
- Traumatic, e.g. after block dissection of lymphatics

also called the French (Fr) gauge system (to calculate the diameter, divide by π!). A size of 10 Fr is small and a size of 22 Fr is large. The usual size used for males is 14 or 16 Fr. The catheters have standard lengths, male catheters being about twice as long as female catheters.

Male Urethral Catheterisation

Retract the foreskin if the penis is not circumcised, use the aseptic technique (clean the area with antiseptic, one hand holding the penis and the other holding the cotton wool with forceps, after which the region is draped), instil anaesthetic gel into the urethra and introduce the catheter fully into the urethra (the penis is usually held vertically or at 45°). Once urine drains, inflate the balloon and connect the catheter to either a free drainage bag or an hourly measuring urine bag. Never inflate the balloon unless you are sure the catheter is in the bladder, with urine seen passing through the catheter. Return the foreskin to prevent a paraphimosis. Note the residual volume of urine and send the specimen of urine for bacteriology. The complications of urethral catheterisation include local trauma, introduction of infection, urethritis and stricture formation.

Some centres advocate the need for routine antibiotic cover for this procedure (usually one dose of gentamycin 80 mg intramuscularly); others feel this is unnecessary. In certain situations antibiotics are essential, for example if the patient has a metal prosthesis such as a hip replacement or if the patient has a heart murmur, since infection in these patients could be disastrous.

Suprapubic Catheters (SPCs)

Suprapubic catheters are used when urethral catheterisation is not possible (e.g. urethral stricture) or is inappropriate, such as when urethral trauma is suspected (pelvic injury with a high-riding prostate). Be aware, however, that suprapubic catheterisation is a dangerous procedure, especially if the patient has had previous lower abdominal surgery. There are many types of SPCs, and they can either be specially manufactured SPCs or inserted using a special introducer such as the Add-a-Cath; alternatively a normal Foley catheter can be used. The Add-a-Cath has a plastic sheath around a sharp-ended trocar. The catheter is inserted into the bladder in the midline about 5 cm above the symphysis pubis. Prior to inserting an SPC there must be no doubt that the bladder is palpable. Urine should be aspirated through a green needle on a syringe prior to attempting SPC insertion. If there is any doubt an ultrasound should be performed. The plastic sheath around the introducer can be zipped down and torn off to allow the whole sheath to be removed once the catheter is in the bladder. The only way to understand this properly is to ask a urologist to show you the actual catheter.

HAEMATURIA

Haematuria can be a finding on urine analysis (microscopic haematuria) or when the patient complains of passing red urine (macroscopic or frank haematuria). Over 35% of patients with frank haematuria have a urological malignancy. Indeed, if you ever see a patient with frank haematuria you should immediately be thinking about renal cell carcinoma (RCC) or bladder cancer.

Haematuria can be due to general or localised causes. The local causes can be bleeding anywhere along the urinary tract – the kidneys, ureters, bladder, prostate or urethra. At any of these sites the bleeding may be due to infections (tuberculosis (TB), schistosomiasis or urinary tract infection (UTI)), stones, trauma or tumours. Renal diseases such as glomerulonephritis also cause haematuria. The general causes include bleeding disorders, leukaemias, haemoglobinopathies and sickle cell disease. These are relatively rare and a local cause must always be excluded. Also note that starting anticoagulants can result in uncovering a local bleeding source. In your history you should elicit the following points:

- Is the blood definitely in the urine and not from the vagina or rectum?
- Is it true haematuria? There are many other causes of red urine, including drugs (e.g. rifampicin, nitrofurantoin), foods such as beetroot, and systemic disease such as porphyrias or rhabdomyolysis.
- Is the haematuria associated with loin pain or pain on passing urine (dysuria)? Pain usually implies stones or infections, whereas painless

- ○ Poor stream
- ○ Intermittent flow and terminal dribbling
- ○ Incomplete emptying (feeling like you need to go again straight-away (*pis-en-deux*), also associated with bladder diverticulae)
- • Irritative symptoms
- ○ Frequency
- ○ Urgency (and urge incontinence)
- ○ Nocturia (needing to get up more than once at night)

The aetiology of the irritative symptoms is poorly understood. These symptoms may be secondary to BPH but can also be a feature of intravesical pathology, such as bladder cancer, UTIs and stones.

The complications of BOO include UTI as a result of urinary stasis, formation of bladder calculi, hydronephrosis and subsequent renal impairment, and acute (painful) and chronic (painless) urinary retention.

BENIGN PROSTATIC HYPERPLASIA (BPH)

The prostate is a capsulated fibromuscular gland, which measures approximately $4 \times 3 \times 2$ cm and normally weighs about 15 g. As the male gets older the gland enlarges, especially in the transitional zone (in contrast to cancer, which affects the peripheral part of the gland). The symptoms are those listed under BOO. Patients must always be asked how much bother their symptoms cause.

The abdomen should be examined to exclude urinary retention. On rectal examination the normal prostate has a smooth surface and there is a palpable midline sulcus. In BPH the normal findings are present but the gland is enlarged. The size and consistency should be noted.

Investigations

Urine should be tested using a dipstick and sent for microscopy and culture. Send blood for U&E to assess renal function. Prostate-specific antigen (PSA) is a protein produced by prostatic acinar cells (both normal and cancerous, although cancerous cells produce about ten times as much). The level of PSA in the blood increases as the prostate increases in size (both in BPH and cancer). The PSA also increases with age. The normal PSA is less than 4 ng/ml at the age of 65 but the normal value increases with age. The higher the PSA the greater the chance of cancer being present. (However, it can be raised markedly with BPH or with a UTI.) If the PSA is high and remains high when rechecked or clinically the prostate is suspicious, then a transrectal ultrasound and biopsy of the prostate can be performed. Patients should be carefully counselled before having their PSA tested.

A urine flow test is performed. This involves passing urine onto a flow meter which generates a graph of urinary volume (ml) against time (s). An ultrasound of the urinary tract is usually performed to assess the residual bladder volume and to look for upper tract dilatation, which may result if the obstruction is severe.

More invasive investigations might include a cystoscopy if a urethral stricture or bladder calculus is suspected or if irritative symptoms predominate. Urodynamic (bladder pressure) studies can be performed for complex cases.

A voiding diary is helpful in seeing how much bother the symptoms cause the patient.

Management

If the symptoms are mild and do not bother the patient, then a policy of watchful waiting may be adopted, with a review in the clinic to see if the symptoms have changed. Approximately 65% of patients will either not improve or get worse.

As long as there is no evidence of complications of bladder outflow obstruction, such as hydronephrosis, recurrent UTIs or urinary retention, treatment is a choice between surgical and medical options, depending on symptom severity and patient preference.

Medical treatment involves the use of α_1-adrenoreceptor blockers such as tamsulosin, prazosin and alfuzosin, which relax the prostatic smooth muscle, increasing urinary flow, and help with the obstructive symptoms. Side effects from these drugs are uncommon but they can cause postural hypotension. 5-α-reductase inhibitors such as finasteride (which block the conversion of testosterone to the more active dihydrotestosterone, the hormone important in developing BPH) have been used but are of doubtful efficacy except in the very large prostate.

Surgical treatment involves removing the obstructing part of the prostate.

Transurethral resection of the prostate (TURP) is the most frequently performed operation for this condition, and the second most common operation (after cataract surgery) performed on men over 60. The patient is placed in a lithotomy position and a resectoscope, passed through the urethra, is used under direct vision to remove the prostate piece by piece, using cutting diathermy. The chippings are sent for histology.

Diathermy is also used to stop any bleeding. A three-way catheter is inserted postoperatively to irrigate the bladder until the fluid is no longer heavily blood-stained. This stops any clots from forming and blocking the catheter. The procedure can be performed with green light (KTP) or holmium laser.

Complications of TURP can be general and specific, early and late, etc.

Early complications include septic shock, bleeding and transurethral syndrome. Transurethral (TUR) syndrome is uncommon and is, like water intoxication, thought to be due to absorption of hypotonic irrigation fluids during the TURP. (Saline cannot be used because it limits the use of diathermy.) It usually occurs during a particularly long and difficult TURP with significant bleeding. The problems include electrolyte imbalances (especially hyponatraemia), haemolysis and fluid overload, and if brain oedema occurs the patient can become confused, have a fit and lose consciousness. Treatment is difficult but essentially involves fluid restriction, diuretics and close observation.

Late complications include secondary haemorrhage, urethral strictures, impotence, recurrent prostatic regrowth and recurrent symptoms. It is essential, when consenting the patient, that he knows that 65–85% of cases will develop retrograde ejaculation (sperm flows into the bladder on orgasm and hence the patient becomes infertile). Some urologists believe that impotence might occur in up to 3–5% of patients postoperatively, although this is debatable. TURP is the gold standard treatment of BPH. As so many men develop BPH, a day case procedure is being sought which will be as effective as TURP. Newer methods for treating BPH include microwave therapy, laser prostatectomy, radiofrequency ablation and prostatic stents. (Find out which technique is used at your hospital.) Open prostatectomy (retropubic or transvesical) is only performed nowadays for very large prostates where the gland is larger than 100 g and TURP would take too long, leading to a high risk of TUR syndrome developing.

UROLOGICAL CANCERS

Carcinoma of the Prostate

The presentation of prostate cancer has changed dramatically in the past 10–15 years, particularly since PSA measurement became available. Whereas previously 70% of cases of prostatic cancer presented late with advanced disease (such as bony metastases), nowadays a high percentage are found in the early stages due to PSA testing of men with BPH or asymptomatic men having a routine health check.

The symptoms can be those of BPH and it can be difficult to differentiate between carcinoma of the prostate and BPH. Carcinoma of the prostate can be diagnosed histologically after TURP for what was thought to be benign disease, when the prostatic chippings are seen under the microscope. However, this is now much less common than it used to be with the use of PSA and prostate biopsy. It is an adenocarcinoma arising in the peripheral zone of the gland (which is also the functional part of the gland). The aetiology is unknown.

On rectal examination the prostate may feel enlarged and "craggy" or a hard nodule may be palpable. The normal midline sulcus may be lost. Investigations depend on the patient's age and his symptoms. If the PSA is raised or clinically the prostate is suspicious, a transrectal ultrasound and biopsy of the prostate should be performed. If a malignancy is diagnosed, the staging procedures include a bone scan and a magnetic resonance imaging (MRI) scan of the abdomen and pelvis, and a set of liver function tests. If the patient has symptoms of bladder outflow obstruction, then as well as investigating the prostate cancer it is also necessary to perform an ultrasound and urine flow tests, as you would when assessing BPH.

The stages of prostatic carcinoma are as follows (via the TNM system; outline of the "T" component of staging):

- T0: No primary tumour identifiable
- T1: Tumour identified incidentally at TURP or with raised PSA
- T2: Palpable tumour without extracapsular extension
- T3: Spread beyond capsule; mobile tumour
- T4: Fixed or locally invasive tumour

Treatment

In early prostate cancer, treatment with curative intent can be offered. Radical prostatectomy performed laparoscopically, with robotic assistance or by open surgery, radical radiotherapy or brachytherapy (the placement of radioactive seeds within the prostate) are performed in men under 70 years with a life expectancy of at least ten years. The best method of treating early prostate cancer is not established and the treatment should be individualised to the patient's circumstances. Many of these treatments have significant complications including impotence and incontinence. Many patients nowadays have read about the different treatments available on the Internet and may have an opinion about what treatment they would like.

Prostate cancer is driven by androgens (testosterone), so in patients with metastatic or locally advanced disease the main aim of treatment is to decrease androgen activity. This is achieved by medical or surgical castration. Medical castration can be achieved by luteinising hormone-releasing hormone (LHRH) agonists such as goserelin (Zoladex), which is administered as a trimonthly subcutaneous injection, or oral antiandrogens such as flutamide or cyproterone. The patients are followed up in the clinic and PSA measurements are used to assess response. Mean survival once metastases are present is a little over 2.5 years. TURP can be performed if obstructive symptoms are present, although some of the obstructive symptoms may resolve with hormone treatment.

There is no national screening for prostate cancer. There are several problems regarding prostate cancer screening. The disease is very common, but in many it does not affect the patient during his life (more than

50% of men over 75 have microfoci at postmortem). An ideal test needs to be found and the best way of treating early prostate cancer needs to be identified. A method of identifying which patients with early prostate cancer will go on to develop metastases is also needed. Until some of these problems are resolved, screening for prostate cancer is regarded by some as inappropriate, particularly as the transrectal biopsy itself can cause complications, particularly urinary sepsis.

Carcinoma of the Bladder

In Britain almost all bladder cancers (98%) are transitional cell carcinomas (TCCs), the remainder being squamous cell carcinomas or adenocarcinomas. In countries with endemic schistosomiasis, squamous cell carcinoma is more common. The aetiology of TCC is unknown, although occupational exposure to chemicals such as aromatic amines and aniline dyes has been implicated as carcinogenic. TCC was the first disease for which industrial compensation was awarded. Smoking increases the risk fourfold (nitrosamines are found in cigarette smoke!). Squamous cell carcinomas are associated with calculi and infections such as schistosomiasis. Adenocarcinomas are associated with persistent urachal remnants (an embryological remnant of the communication between the umbilicus and the bladder).

Carcinoma of the bladder affects males more than females and usually presents with painless haematuria (about 15% present with recurrent UTIs). Urine cytology may identify abnormal cells in the urine, but the diagnosis is usually made by cystoscopy. When seeing a patient with haematuria, always think of cancer first.

Staging is by the TNM system (outline of the "T" component of staging):

- Ta: Confined to mucosa
- T1: Tumour invading the lamina propria
- T2: Muscle is involved
- T3: Perivesical fat involved
- T4: Invasion beyond the bladder into adjacent organs or fixed to the pelvic side wall

The pathologist also grades them histologically into Grades I–III. Grade I means well-differentiated and Grade III poorly differentiated.

Superficial Bladder Cancers

These can be low-grade or high-grade Ta or T1 tumours. The low-grade superficial tumours are usually exophytic papillary TCCs and about 15% will progress to invasive cancers over ten years. Treatment is by cystoscopy and endoscopic resection or diathermy. If no obvious lesion is seen on cystoscopy, multiple biopsies should be taken to exclude carcinoma *in situ* (CIS). High-grade (G3) T1 tumours are aggressive and thus need aggressive treatment. Following resection and diathermy, intravesical chemotherapy (e.g. mitomycin) is given to reduce the likelihood of recurrences. Patients are usually followed up every few months with regular cystoscopies to watch for recurrences. CIS behaves like a high-grade TCC and therefore also requires aggressive treatment. Intravesical immunotherapy with BCG can be used to prevent progression of CIS.

Invasive Bladder Cancers

Bladder cancers that have invaded the muscle are treated most commonly by radical cystectomy and formation of an ileal conduit or creation of a neobladder out of small bowel (usually a length of ileum). An ileal conduit results in a stoma. Formation of a neobladder requires highly complex surgery with a high complication rate and is reserved for patients who are young, motivated and with a high chance of cure from the cystectomy. Cystectomy may be performed in the presence of locally advanced or metastatic disease for intractable bladder symptoms.

RENAL TUMOURS

Malignant tumours can be primary or secondary, although secondary tumours in the kidney are unusual. The primary tumours which usually affect those over 50 years old can arise from the kidney substance itself, and are called renal cell carcinomas, or from the lining of the collecting system (in the pelvis or ureters), and are called transitional cell cancers.

Other tumours include Wilms' tumour (which affect children) and lymphomas. Cysts are very common in the kidney and simple cysts, which display no thickening or calcification in the cyst wall, are completely benign.

Renal Cell Carcinomas (RCCs)

Renal cell carcinomas account for more than 80% of renal tumours. These are renal adenocarcinomas. (In the past it was thought that they arose from the adrenal rests within the kidney, and hence their old name was "hypernephroma".) They actually arise in the renal tubules and are also known as clear cell carcinomas, since the cells appear clear. (They are large, with lots of lipid in the cytoplasm.)

The aetiology is unknown but there is an increased incidence in tobacco smokers. As RCCs grow they become encapsulated by a rim of normal kidney tissue. They can present with haematuria or with pain (due to pressure effects on local structures and nerves). The classic presentation of an RCC is therefore the triad of pain, haematuria and a renal mass, although this triad is rare and usually the patient has only one or two of these symptoms. RCCs can grow along the renal vein and up the inferior vena cava, and metastases are therefore usually blood-borne and commonly go to the lungs (cannonball metastases), bone (pathological fractures), brain, etc. They may present with symptoms due to the production of hormones such as erythropoietin (polycythaemia) or parathyroid hormone-like substance (hypercalcaemia). Although much loved by the older textbooks, these presentations are in fact quite rare. Nowadays about 50% of RCCs are found incidentally in patients having an ultrasound scan or CT scan for unrelated symptoms.

On examination a mass may be palpable in the loin. A common question is, "How do you differentiate a kidney from a spleen?" The kidney is ballotable (place one hand on the abdomen and the other in the renal angle, raise the hand in the renal angle and keep the other hand still; if you feel a mass touch your upper hand, you have balloted a kidney), it moves vertically down on inspiration and finally it is resonant to percussion (due to the overlying colon). The spleen, on the other hand, has a notch and moves towards the right iliac fossa on inspiration and is dull to percussion.

If an RCC obstructs the renal vein, a varicocoele can result on the left. If you see a varicocoele in the left scrotum, think of an RCC, since the testicular vein on the left drains into the renal vein (it enters the IVC directly on the right). Only 1% of renal tumours, however, present with a varicocoele.

Diagnosis is usually made on ultrasound, showing a solid mass arising from the kidney. A CT scan is necessary for staging the disease. The other kidney must be checked not only to make sure it is present and functioning, but also because the disease may be bilateral. Treatment is usually by radical nephrectomy (removing the kidney, surrounding fat within Gerota's fascia, with or without the adrenal gland). Partial nephrectomy can be considered if the tumour is small (<4 cm) or if the patient has a single kidney or poor renal function. Renal cell carcinomas have proved themselves to be resistant to chemotherapy and radiotherapy. There is some evidence supporting the use of immunotherapy with interferons in advanced disease but the benefits are marginal. More recently, tyrosine kinase inhibitors such as sunitinib have been shown to have a role in treating patients with metastatic RCC.

Pelviureteric Tumours

These are the same as the transitional cell carcinomas of the bladder, although they account for less than 20% of renal tumours (whereas TCCs account for almost all bladder tumours). They usually present with haematuria. Diagnosis is made by IVU showing a filling defect or CT IVU. Treatment is usually nephrectomy plus removal of the ureter on that side (nephroureterectomy). Follow-up must include regular cystoscopies to look for tumours in the bladder (50% of patients will subsequently develop bladder tumours).

Wilms' Tumours

A Wilms' tumour (nephroblastoma) contains a bizarre variety of cell and tissue components derived from the mesoderm (for example, as well as kidney substance they may contain fat, cartilage and bone). This is the commonest intra-abdominal tumour in under-10s, with a peak incidence in those aged

2–3. It usually presents with a mass, and diagnosis is by ultrasound, CT or MRI. About 10% are bilateral. It is an aggressive, rapidly growing tumour that often metastasises to the lungs. Treatment is usually radical nephrectomy. Chemotherapy is sometimes given postoperatively, depending on the stage. If the tumour is caught early enough, survival is high.

TESTICULAR TUMOURS

Accounting for less than 2% of male malignancies, these are uncommon (despite being the commonest solid tumours in young men). The incidence is about 7 per 100,000 men. Testicular tumours can be divided into germ-cell and non-germ-cell tumours. Almost all are germ-cell tumours. The germ-cell tumours can be divided into seminomas (40%), non-seminomatous germ-cell tumours or NSGCTs (10%) (also called teratomas) and mixed (40%). Rarely, choriocarcinomas and yolk sac tumours are seen (these are types of NSGCTs).

For finals the most important testicular tumours to know about are the seminomas and teratomas. The peak incidence is at 20–40 years. 2% are bilateral and there is a significantly increased risk in men with undescended testes.

Non-germ-cell tumours include Leydig cell and Sertoli cell tumours and lymphomas. The Leydig cell and Sertoli cell tumours are very rare; however, they can produce oestrogens and androgens, resulting in overvirilisation or feminisation. Lymphomas can occur in the testicle in men in the fifth and sixth decades.

Seminomas arise in the epithelium of the seminiferous tubules, tend to grow slowly and metastasise to regional and para-aortic lymph nodes. (Remember that the lymphatics usually follow the venous drainage and the testicular veins drain towards the IVC and not to the groin.) NSGCTs arise from all three germ-cell layers, can be more aggressive and carry a poorer prognosis than seminomas. They are subdivided histologically, depending on whether the tumour is well-differentiated, moderately differentiated or undifferentiated. The more undifferentiated carry a poorer prognosis. They metastasise via the blood and the lymphatics and most of them secrete β-human-chorionic-gonadotropin (βHCG) and α-fetoprotein (AFP), which are used as tumour markers.

The staging of testicular tumours is as follows:

- Stage I: Tumour confined to testis
- Stage II: Involvement of lymph nodes below diaphragm
- Stage III: Lymph nodes above diaphragm involved
- Stage IV: Extralymphatic spread

The tumours usually present as a painless testicular mass, although they can present with a secondary hydrocoele or a painful lump (10% present with pain). They may be misdiagnosed initially as epididymo-orchitis. On examination you should look for evidence of lymphatic spread (abdominal, supraclavicular and chest).

A common exam question concerns how to examine a scrotum. You should always ask yourself four questions: Can I get above it? (You should be able to get above a testicular lesion, but not a hernia.) Is the lump in the testis or is it separate? Does it transilluminate? Is the testis tender? A hard mass in the testis, which you can get above and which does not transilluminate, is likely to represent a testicular tumour.

An ultrasound can be performed to see if a scrotal lump is connected with the testis and if it is solid or cystic. A solid lump suggests malignancy. Blood for serum AFP (never raised in seminomas) and βHCG should be sent. To stage the disease a CT scan of the chest, abdomen and pelvis is performed. Treatment starts with an orchidectomy via a groin incision. The reason for the groin incision is threefold: to allow the cord to be clamped before mobilising the testicle, to prevent seeding the scrotal skin and to allow the incision to be within the radiotherapy field. The testis is then brought out and examined. If the lump appears malignant (or a frozen section is performed to confirm the diagnosis histologically), then it is excised together with the spermatic cord. Further treatment depends on the tumour type, and its stage and grade. Tumour markers should again be sent after orchidectomy; if they are still high after surgery this indicates the presence of residual disease.

Seminomas are very radiosensitive. Radiotherapy is usually given both to the groin and to the abdominal lymph nodes. Stage IV tumours are usually given chemotherapy initially, although they are rare (as seminomas usually present earlier than teratomas). Teratomas are less sensitive to radiotherapy, and combination chemotherapy (for example, bleomycin, etoposide and cisplatin) is usually given at the start.

The prognosis for Stage I seminomas and teratomas is extremely good (96–100% five-year survival). For Stage IV disease, five-year survival is 55–75%, depending on the tumour and the tumour bulk. Any recurrence following initial treatment is likely to occur within the first 18–24 months and close surveillance is therefore very important over this period, with repeat CT scanning and measurement of tumour markers, initially every six weeks and then every three months.

OTHER CONDITIONS OF THE TESTES

Hydrocoele

This is the presence of fluid around the testis between the tunica vaginalis and the tunica albuginea (Figure 14.1). The condition can be primary or secondary. Primary (idiopathic) hydrocoeles, which make up the vast majority, develop slowly and can become large and tense. They are commonest in the over-40 age group, although they can occur in children. If you recall your embryology, the testis descends from the abdomen, taking a layer of peritoneum with it called the processus vaginalis. Normally the processus vaginalis closes, removing the communication between the abdomen and the scrotum; however, if it remains patent, peritoneal fluid can fill the sac, causing an infantile hydrocoele. (If bowel contents enter the sac, then this is an infantile hernia; treatment of the infantile hydrocoele is the same as that for an infantile hernia, that is, to close off the processus vaginalis.) Primary hydrocoeles develop in adults in the absence of a patent processus, the tunica vaginalis producing excessive fluid for unknown reasons. Secondary hydrocoeles are usually secondary to trauma, infection or malignancy and tend to develop more rapidly.

On examination you can get above the swelling (which has a smooth surface), the testis is usually impalpable and it transilluminates brilliantly. An ultrasound should be performed to look at the testis. A small hydrocoele may not need treatment if the patient is not bothered by it. Larger

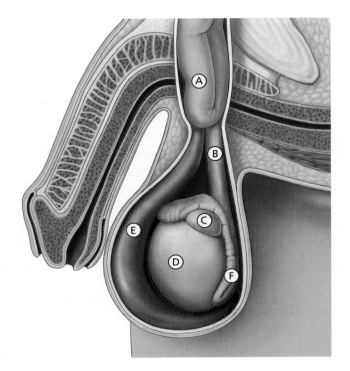

Figure 14.1. Testicular lumps: (A) indirect inguinal hernia, (B) spermatic cord, (C) epididymal cyst, (D) testis, (E) hydrocoele, (F) epididymis.

hydrocoeles can be tapped but the fluid (which is straw-coloured) will invariably return. Definitive surgical treatment involves either plicating the tunica vaginalis (Lord's repair) or inverting the sac (Jaboulay's repair).

Epididymo-orchitis

This is inflammation of the testis and epididymis due to infection. The young are more susceptible to viral infections (e.g. mumps), the old to bacterial infections (e.g. *Escherichia coli* following a UTI) and the sexually active to chlamydial and gonococcal infection.

The typical presentation is acute onset of severe testicular pain. The patient may feel unwell with fever, have urethral discharge and symptoms of a UTI. Pain may be referred to the right iliac fossa. On examination the testis is tender, red and warm. You can often feel a markedly swollen epididymis separate from the testicle. If you place your hand under the scrotum and elevate it, this sometimes relieves the pain of epididymo-orchitis, but not of torsion.

Testicular Torsion

This can affect any age but is most common between the ages of 12 and 27; it can occur, rarely, in neonates. There is a higher incidence in undescended testes. It is a urological emergency, as the testis will infarct within hours if the torsion is not treated. The testis twists within the tunica vaginalis and the blood supply is compromised. It usually presents with severe pain of very sudden onset and there are invariably no symptoms of a UTI. In contrast, a patient with epididymo-orchitis usually has a longer history of symptoms and may have urethritis with burning pain on micturition. On examination, if the testis lies horizontally or is retracted compared to the other side, this could be indicative of a torsion.

An MSU should be tested using a dipstick and sent urgently for microscopy, as this may help in cases where infection is likely. However, if you are in any doubt, then surgical exploration is essential. If you explore it and it is an infection, no harm is done, but if you treat a torsion conservatively the testicle will die. When you are exploring a testicle for torsion, the patient must always be warned of the possibility of orchidectomy if the testicle has infarcted. At the time of surgery both testicles are fixed (with a suture) to the scrotal wall to ensure they cannot twist in the future. Doppler ultrasound is quite good at showing the integrity of the arterial blood flow to the testis, but should not be relied upon and should not delay surgical exploration.

RENAL COLIC

Stones may form at any level of the urinary tract. Symptoms depend on the site of stone impaction, its size and any sequelae. The pain most commonly associated with ureteric stones is due to the peristalsis and dilatation proximal to the obstruction. The size of the stone is not correlated with the amount of pain, as a large staghorn calculus of the renal pelvis may be painless while a tiny stone in the ureter may be agonising. The classic story is sudden onset of severe pain that makes the patient writhe about in agony, unable to get comfortable (in contrast with the pain of peritonism, where the patient lies still). The patient is sweaty, nauseous and may vomit. A stone in the ureter usually causes pain which starts in the loin and radiates down into the groin. There may also be pain in the scrotum or labia. The pain from a stone in the midureter may mimic appendicitis on the right and diverticulitis on the left.

Most urinary tract calculi are calcium stones (80%) complexed with oxalate (35%), phosphate (3%) or mixed oxalate and phosphate crystals (40%). Others include struvite (magnesium ammonium phosphate), cystine, urate and xanthine. They usually form when there is a high concentration of solutes in the urine, especially in dehydration. Most stone formers excrete excessive amounts of calcium in their urine, and are called hypercalciuric. There may be a familial tendency and calcium stones may rarely be associated with hyperparathyroidism, renal tubular acidosis and medullary sponge kidney. Triple phosphate (struvite) stones are associated with UTIs, especially *Proteus*, which breaks down urea to form ammonia, resulting in alkaline urine which precipitates these stones. In contrast, acid urine tends to precipitate the calcium oxalate and urate-containing stones.

90% of renal stones are radio-opaque (urate stones are radiolucent), in contrast to gallstones, where 90% are radiolucent. Examination is usually normal, although the patient may have tenderness in the renal angle, especially on percussion, which indicates retroperitoneal inflammation. A urine dipstick should reveal haematuria (in over 90% of cases) and this should be confirmed by microscopy. If the urine shows no blood you should be thinking of alternative diagnoses. Note that renal colic is not a diagnosis; it is a simply a symptom of ureteric obstruction which may be caused by a stone but could be due to an aortic aneurysm, TCC of the ureter, retroperitoneal lymph nodes, etc. Other causes of pain mimicking ureteric colic include an abdominal aortic aneurysm, appendicitis, pyelonephritis, diverticulitis and gynaecological causes.

Analgesia should be given once the diagnosis is suspected. The pain from ureteric colic is usually alleviated by non-steroidal anti-inflammatory agents but may require opiates. Preliminary evaluation is with a CT KUB (with no contrast) or an IVU by the casualty doctor. You should familiarise yourself with both these investigations.

A CT KUB is a rapid investigation which is the investigation of choice where available. Some centres still use IVU initially. When performing an IVU, a baseline KUB X-ray is taken first. You should know the normal course of the ureters. They start at the renal pelvis, which lies at the level of L1 or L2 (look for the 12th rib, which is joined to T12, and go down one vertebra). They travel down from here along the line of the transverse processes towards the sacroiliac joint or SIJ (where they cross over the iliac vessels). At this point they travel backwards towards the ischial spines and then forwards into the bladder. The common sites for obstruction to occur are the pelviureteric junction, the SIJ, where the ureter crosses over the iliac vessels, and the vesicoureteric junction (VUJ). Remember that phleboliths (calcification in veins) are common in this region, but they are usually multiple, more rounded and have a radiolucent centre. A Venflon is inserted and the radio-opaque contrast is injected into the arm. A film is taken after 5 min and another postmicturition. If there is any abnormality on the IVU, then a delayed film after about 1 h is usually taken. Further films should be taken until contrast is seen down to the level of obstruction. Request films at 1, 2, 4, 8 and 24 h if necessary. In the normal kidney, contrast is seen flowing towards the bladder. The ureter is a hollow tube that peristalses six times a minute. Students often get confused because they see some contrast in the ureter and then see what looks like a stricture and think this must be a block. Actually, this simply represents a wave of peristalsis and is normal. If there is a block, what you see is a standing column of contrast above the stone. The renal pelvis may be dilated and there may be blunting of the calyces. If there is complete obstruction on one side you may see a dense nephrogram (the kidney outline is visibly radio-opaque), with no contrast entering the ureter.

Nowadays, instead of an IVU, an unenhanced CT scan may be used to image the renal tract when stone disease is expected. This is safe in patients who are allergic to iodine. (The contrast used for the IVU contains iodine.) Diabetics on metformin have to stop taking their medication 24 h prior to having an IVU. Asthmatics may require steroid cover for contrast imaging.

Varicocoeles

A varicocoele is an abnormal dilatation of the testicular veins (essentially varicose veins of the testicle) caused by venous reflux down the gonadal veins. They most often occur on the left side (80–90%) for anatomical reasons, as the left gonadal vein arises directly from the longer left renal vein. They are usually asymptomatic and are described as like "a bag of worms" in the scrotum on examination. They are more prominent on standing — so ask the patient to stand if you are examining for a varicocoele or if you suspect one. Occasionally the patient may complain of aching or heaviness in the scrotum on standing but their main importance is that they are thought to be associated with male infertility, possibly due to chronically raising the temperature of the testicle. A rare cause, but sometimes asked about, is blockage of the left renal vein by a renal tumour causing reflux down the gonadal vein. Most varicocoeles can be managed conservatively but if required they can be treated by surgical ligation or radiological techniques such as embolisation to block the veins responsible. Repair of a varicocoele in order to improve fertility is non-evidence-based and doubts exist as to whether it is worthwhile, but it is still sometimes performed for that reason.

PAEDIATRIC UROLOGY

At birth, adhesions are present between the glans and the foreskin (prepuce). The prepuce normally becomes retractile by the age of two. Sometimes the parents notice the prepuce "ballooning" when the child micturates due to urine collecting in the space between the foreskin and glans, before escaping through the narrow opening. This is normal and the parents should be reassured.

Phimosis

Phimosis, a narrowing of the opening of the foreskin, can be the result of recurrent balanitis. It is usually treated by circumcision. (A paraphimosis is a swelling of the glans as a result of a tight foreskin being retracted and not replaced. This can occur after catheterisation or erection. The tight foreskin blocks the venous return and the glans becomes oedematous and swollen. This is usually treated by reducing the oedema with compression, squeezing the foreskin and glans. The glans is then pressed in whilst flipping the foreskin forwards to its normal position.)

Hypospadias

This is an abnormal position of the urethral opening, due to failure of normal development. The urethra can open anywhere on the ventral surface (undersurface) of the penis. Repair is usually carried out by paediatric surgeons.

Undescended Testes

The testes drop into the scrotum in weeks 28–34 of foetal development. They sometimes fail to descend fully, resulting in undescended testes. All neonates should be examined at birth to determine if the testes are in the scrotum. In 80% of cases the undescended testis is palpable in the inguinal canal. If the testis is palpable in the inguinal canal or at the top of the scrotum, orchidopexy is performed (the testis is fixed in the scrotum, usually by mobilising the testis and placing it between the dartos muscle and the skin). This should be done by the age of 18 months, to prevent damage to the testis (spontaneous descent is rare after one year). After the age of two, the testis is likely to be damaged and may become incapable of spermatogenesis.

Complete absence of the testis is uncommon (check notes to see if present at birth check), and if it is not palpable it should be assumed to be intra-abdominal and an MRI or laparoscopy may be needed to locate it. If an undescended testicle presents after puberty, many urologists would advocate location and removal of the testicle because of the risk of malignant change.

15

ORTHOPAEDICS

Peter Smitham and Andy Goldberg

In this chapter we have tried to cover the most important subjects that you need to know for the final examination. As much as possible we have tried to discuss principles rather than list every type of injury and fracture, because these principles can then be applied to many different clinical situations.

You should especially know how to examine the hand, hip, knee and shoulder with fluency and should practise these examinations on patients and on friends before the exam, so that they become second nature. Orthopaedic surgeons have in the past been stereotyped as using four-letter words and so it may come as no surprise that the orthopaedic examination can be summarised by the following words: look, feel, move and X-ray. It is really difficult to learn specialised examination tests from a book and so we urge you to ask an orthopaedic consultant or registrar to demonstrate the examinations to you as well.

Always ask the patient if they mind you examining them and whether they have any pain or tenderness (in a similar way to checking your mirrors in a driving test, make sure the examiners note that you have done so). Also observe the patient's face for pain during the examination, because hurting your patient is one of the biggest errors you can make in the exam.

Remember you should always examine the normal side first and then use this as a comparison for the abnormal or painful side. Also, in order to be seen to be thorough, you should always offer to examine the joint above and below the one you are asked to do. Finish off each examination by saying you would like to perform a neurological and vascular examination as well.

EXAMINATION OF THE HIP

Quick Notes on the Hip

- Pain arising from the hip joint is often felt in the groin or anterior thigh, and sometimes it is referred down to the knee. If the pain is predominantly in the back of the hip, it is usually referred from the lumbar spine. It is true to say that pain is usually referred distally, and so a knee pain may be coming from the hip and a hip pain may be coming from the back, etc.

Students often get worried about the correct order to examine a joint. The fact is that no order is necessarily correct and often the order of examination will differ depending on the circumstances. For example, an elderly lady seen in casualty after a fall will be assessed supine on a trolley, whereas a young patient may be standing and so you could choose to examine gait initially. To examine the hips properly, both legs need to be exposed (i.e. undress the patient to the underwear).

If circumstances allow, start the examination by getting the patient to stand in front of you. Observe for any gross pelvic obliquity, any knee malalignment and for any problems with the feet. Ask the patient to walk towards you and observe their gait. If they have a stick, try to observe their gait with and without the stick if possible. For ease of explanation we will discuss gait at the end of this section.

Then ask the patient to get onto the couch and observe how easy or difficult that is for them. With the patient supine, on inspection look at the attitude (or posture) of the limbs; for example, is one leg shortened or externally rotated compared to the other? Look for any obvious scars but do not forget to check the buttocks, as a scar centred over the greater trochanter extending over the buttock could indicate previous hip replacement (these are often hidden underneath a patient's pants and so you must check underneath them). Also check for swelling or wasting of the quadriceps, glutei or hamstrings. Inspect the legs for signs of venous or arterial disease (which will be important if an operation is being considered) and examine for any leg length discrepancy.

To do this, you should differentiate between real shortening (loss of bone length) and apparent shortening (e.g. due to a tilted pelvis). First, try to position the pelvis so that the anterior superior iliac spines (ASIS) are at the same horizontal level.

On palpation measure the distance from the ASIS to the medial malleolus on each side (true length) and the distance from a fixed point such as the xiphisternum (or umbilicus) to the medial malleolus (apparent length). The apparent length will differ from the true length if the pelvis is tilted (pelvic obliquity). Feel the bony contours, including the greater trochanter, the ASIS, the iliac crests and the pubic rami.

Test movement passively and actively. Normal ranges for the hip are as follows: flexion (0–130°), extension (usually in a prone position, 0–10°), abduction (0–45°), adduction (0–30°), external rotation (0–45°) and internal rotation (0–20°). Rotation can be tested with the hips flexed (i.e. knees bent to 90°) or in extension. In flexion, put one hand on the knee and the other on the foot — remember that external rotation brings the foot medially. To test adduction the limb is crossed over the opposite limb. Power should be recorded for each muscle group. One problem with the hip is that limitation of movement can be obscured by movement of the pelvis and hence a gross limitation of extension can be masked by arching the back into excessive lordosis. Therefore, when describing the range of motion, always comment on any fixed flexion deformities first. You can use Thomas's test to check for this — fully flex the two hips simultaneously to obliterate the lumbar lordosis (you can place one hand under the lower back to confirm this). Whilst holding one leg in this position, ask the patient to straighten the other leg as fully as possible. The angle between the thigh and the bed is the fixed flexion deformity. Repeat the test on the other side. The commonest cause of a fixed flexion deformity is capsular fibrosis and osteophytes seen in osteoarthritis (OA).

The function and stability of the hip can be assessed by Trendelenburg's test. Ask the patient to stand on one leg by bending at the knee (as if they were doing an impression of a pirate with a wooden leg!). The normal pelvis tilts upwards on the unsupported side by contraction of the abductors on the weight-bearing side. A positive Trendelenburg sign occurs when the pelvis droops on the unsupported side — "sound side sags". The causes of a positive test include weakness of the abductors, dislocation or fracture of the hip and in fact any painful condition of the hip.

You must always examine the patient's gait. If the patient is dependent on a walking stick or calliper, then you can ask them to use it. Gait involves all the joints of the lower limb, and it is therefore difficult sometimes to discern the exact cause of an abnormal gait. If the patient limps because of pain, then this is called antalgic gait, whereby the weight-bearing (stance) phase on the affected side is shorter, as the patient tries to avoid putting weight onto this side. The commonest cause is osteoarthritis. If one leg is shorter than the other, this is described as a short-legged gait but the stance phase is not reduced (unless there are coexisting short-legged and antalgic elements). Also observe for any torsional abnormalities by observing the patient's foot progression angle, i.e. whether the foot points in the same direction as the patella.

Incidentally, if you see a case in finals where one leg is smaller or deformed with asymmetrical muscular wasting and sensation is entirely normal, always look around the room for a calliper or cast brace, as polio cases often feature in finals (despite the fact that we see almost no new cases in the developed world!).

EXAMINATION OF THE KNEE

Quick Notes on the Knee

- There are three components to the knee joint: the medial and lateral compartments (each between the femoral condyles and tibial plateau) and the patellofemoral compartment. The joint surfaces are lined by hyaline or articular cartilage (which becomes worn in osteoarthritis). In addition, there are the two C-shaped menisci or shock absorbers that line the medial and lateral compartments. These are not made of hyaline cartilage but instead of fibrocartilage and their roles are to protect the articular cartilage and give extra stability and conformity to the joint. There are two parallel ligaments running in opposite directions at the centre of the knee, which help make it stable, called the cruciate ligaments. The anterior cruciate limits forward translation and internal rotation of the tibia relative to the femur. Similarly, the posterior cruciate stops the tibia moving from backwards relative to the femur. The capsule encloses the knee joint and is strengthened on the medial and lateral sides by the medial and lateral collateral ligaments.

As mentioned above, gait can be tested at the beginning or at the end of the examination — it does not really matter, as long as you remember to test for it and you build a system that you are comfortable using.

Like with the hip, start the examination by getting the patient to stand facing you. Observe the alignment, checking for valgus (knock-knees or genu valgum — deviation of the distal part away from the midline) or varus deformities at the knees. Look at the foot arches to see if they are flattened (pes planus) or high-arched (pes cavus), which can contribute to knee pathology. Then get the patient to face away from you and observe the alignment of the knees from behind and the hindfeet. Then ask the patient to turn 90° and observe for any flexion (or extension) deformities at the knees. Remember to ask the patient to fully extend the knee at this point, otherwise you may falsely assume there is a fixed flexion deformity. Whilst the patient is standing it is useful to look for any scars. Two to three small stab incisions along the joint line may represent an arthroscopy; a large midline incision may represent a total knee replacement; whilst scars off-centre may be due to an old open menisectomy or unicompartmental knee replacement. Posterior scars are often in the shape of a lazy S and most commonly due to vascular surgery.

Then ask the patient to get onto the couch. When they are lying supine, look and measure for quadriceps wasting (which implies lack of use). This ideally should be done at 10 cm from the upper pole of the patella, as this correlates with vastus medialis wasting, which is the first muscle to be affected by disuse. Then observe whether the patellae are symmetrical and for any obvious effusions to the knees (even a small effusion may be noted by the absence of the normal hollow on either side of the patella).

Feel the skin temperature, which is helpful in the knee as the joint is superficial (unlike the hip), always comparing with the opposite side.

Now test for an effusion. To do this, you can use the patella tap or stroke test. To perform the patella tap, compress the suprapatellar pouch with one hand and press down gently on the patella with the fingers of your opposite hand. You should be able to bounce the patella up and down on the fluid, always comparing with the other side. If there is only a small effusion a better test is the stroke test (sometimes known as the swipe test), where you empty the medial compartment by massaging the fluid into the lateral side of the knee. Then apply gentle pressure over the lateral side, just above the patella, and watch the gutter on the medial side. If there is an effusion, the medial gutter will balloon up with the fluid you have pushed over.

Ask the patient to move their leg by lifting it straight into the air (with the knee extended). If the leg is lifted straight then the quadriceps must be working normally. If there is a lag (meaning that the knee bends slightly as it is raised) then this either means that the quadriceps are injured or weak or that there is a fixed flexion deformity. Place the flat of your palm under the ankle and ask the patient to let you take the full weight of the leg. If by doing so the leg straightens fully then you know there is no fixed flexion, whereas if it remains bent then there must be a fixed flexion deformity (the commonest cause being capsular fibrosis/osteophytes in osteoarthritis).

Put your other hand over the knee cap (a right-handed examiner, examining the right leg, would hold the ankle with the right hand and the knee cap with the left hand) and feel for crepitus as the knee is flexed and extended. Crepitus can signify irregular articular surfaces, often found in osteoarthritis or chondromalacia patella. Note the full range of active movement of both legs. A normal knee should be able to flex to about 140°. Now bend the knee to 90° and rest the foot down on the bed. Put both heels together at this point to compare. Palpate along the joint line. Remember that in this position the joint line is angled downwards at about a 45° slant, and so your thumb must feel the joint line which has a spongy consistency (unlike the bone just below it). Feel along the medial joint line and lateral joint line respectively. Tenderness at any point usually indicates meniscal pathology (but remember it could indicate a problem with any of the structures below your finger, i.e. skin, capsule, ligaments or bone).

The popliteal fossa should be examined to exclude a popliteal cyst and a pulsatile popliteal aneurysm. A popliteal cyst is a non-tender fluctuant lump that follows either synovial rupture or herniation. If there is underlying joint pathology such as osteoarthritis, then it is called a Baker's cyst. Do not confuse a popliteal cyst or aneurysm (which are in the midline) with an enlarged semimembranosus bursa, which is on the medial side between the semimembranosus and the medial head of the gastrocnemius and is often more prominent in a straight knee.

There are lots of special tests for the patellofemoral joint which you normally carry out only if the symptoms are suggestive of patellofemoral pathology. They are beyond the scope of this book, so please ask your consultant or registrar to show them to you as they are important pieces of the knowledge you will need to have for finals. You can, however, test the side-to-side movements of the patella. In a normal individual you should be able to feel one third of the undersurface of the patella when moving the patella from side to side. The patella apprehension test is for patellas that have dislocated in the past — when the patella is pushed laterally, the patient becomes anxious, as they might feel like it is going to dislocate.

To test for tears of the collateral ligaments, flex the knee slightly (about 20°) and apply valgus and varus stress to the knee joint to see if there is any laxity. The knee has to be bent slightly because in full extension it normally "locks". If the knee opens up to valgus or varus stress in full extension then you should be concerned about a very serious injury and complete rupture of the ligaments. If the ligaments are tender to palpation but the knee feels stable to stressing, this usually indicates a strain or partial tear rather than a complete tear.

Diagnosis of meniscal pathology is usually made from the history, together with the finding of joint line tenderness. There is something called McMurray's test, which is described in lots of textbooks, but I feel that these descriptions are often far removed from McMurray's original description. The test is not very accurate and can potentially propagate a meniscal tear. In view of this, no further mention is made of this test. You will not fail an exam for not knowing specific tests, although you could fail if you hurt a patient by doing complex tests incorrectly or inappropriately.

of the arc of movement is painful. Pain at the beginning to midrange of movement is usually due to rotator cuff pathology, such as inflammation or a tear of the supraspinatus. Pain at the end of abduction may be due to acromioclavicular osteoarthritis. Observe movement at the glenohumeral joint and of the scapula on both sides. Test also flexion, extension, rotation and adduction (where the arm moves in front of the body). Active rotation is best tested by asking the patient to touch the back of their neck with both hands (external rotation in abduction) and the small of their back (internal rotation). Now passively repeat all of these movements.

Passive rotation is tested with the elbow touching the side of the body and flexed to 90°. Bringing the hand across the body to touch the patient's belly is internal rotation, and away from the body, external rotation. Record the power of each muscle group (using the Medical Research Council grading system, from 1 to 5) and test for any neurovascular deficit.

Test for winging of the scapulae by asking the patient to place their hands out in front of them, pressing against a wall. If the serratus anterior is paralysed, the scapula will protrude like a wing.

There are many special tests for the shoulder; however, you probably just need to know the ones mentioned for the purposes of finals. A terribly rare inherited disorder is craniocleidodysostosis, where there is absence of the clavicles and the patient can bring both shoulders to the midline. This is the sort of rare but interesting case that sometimes turns up in exams, so it is probably worth a mention.

EXAMINATION OF THE HANDS

Quick Notes on the Hands

- The thumb, the index finger and the middle finger are the most important for the functioning of the hand (touch, grip, precise movements), whereas the ring finger and the little finger are more important for grip strength.
- Distal interphalangeal joints = DIPJs, proximal interphalangeal joints = PIPJs and metacarpophalangeal joints = MCPJs.
- Refer to the fingers as the thumb, index, middle, ring and little fingers, not 1, 2, 3, 4 and 5.

- The DIPJs are flexed by the flexor digitorum profundus (inserting into the base of the distal phalanx) and the PIPJs are flexed by the flexor digitorum superficialis (which splits around the profundus and inserts into the base of the middle phalanx).
- The flexor digitorum profundus (FDP) is innervated by both the median and ulnar nerves, usually the median nerve supplying the part that flexes the index and middle fingers, with the ulnar nerve supplying the part that flexes the ring and little fingers.
- The Palmar interossei ADduct the fingers (PAD), whereas the Dorsal interossei ABduct or spread the fingers (DAB).
- The interossei and lumbricals are responsible for flexion at the MCPJs (whilst the PIPJs and DIPJs are extended).
- All of the intrinsic muscles of the hand are supplied by T1 as the ulnar nerve, except the LOAF muscles (see the section on carpal tunnel syndrome), which are supplied by the median nerve.
- Primary osteoarthritis tends to affect the DIPJs (and the PIPJs) whereas rheumatoid arthritis (RA) tends to affect the MCPJs and PIPJs, sparing the DIPJs.

Hands are very commonly seen in finals (usually as a rheumatology case). You may still see a rheumatoid hand in surgical exams although you are more likely to see a nerve injury, Dupuytren's disease, trigger finger or a ganglion. As hand examination is covered well in the rheumatology books, you will simply find a summary of the examination here.

Introduce yourself and ask the patient whether they mind you examining their hands and whether they are painful. If a pillow is available, place it under the hands for comfort.

Inspect the hands, look at the dorsum and then ask the patient to turn their hands over so that you can look at the palms. Observe any scars, palmar erythema, muscle wasting, nail changes or obvious deformities such as Dupuytren's contracture, mallet finger, Boutonniere, swan neck, Z-thumb deformities, Heberden's nodes (which are nodular swellings at the DIPJs, seen in osteoarthritis) and Bouchard's nodes (similar swellings seen at the PIPJs).

Feel the temperature and palpate all of the individual joints (especially the MCPJs), feeling for any synovial or capsular thickening or swelling (indicative of active synovitis). Feel the palm of the hand for thickenings or nodules of the palmar fascia suggestive of early Dupuytren's.

Ask the patient to make a fist and then to touch the thumb to the tip of each finger (opposition). Then test finger abduction and adduction. Test the strength of each of these muscle groups by asking the patient to grasp your finger in a grip and to stop you from pulling your fingers out from between their opposed thumb and little finger. Test resisted abduction by asking the patient to keep their fingers spread against resistance, and resisted adduction by asking them to grip a piece of paper between their adducted fingers as you pull it out (best to hold the paper between your adducted fingers as well, and not between your thumb and index finger — so you are comparing like with like).

Test sensation in the median (the tip of the index finger), radial (the dorsum of the base of the thumb) and ulnar (the tip of the little finger) nerve distributions. As to testing the nerve function in more detail, see the section on nerve injuries at the end of the chapter. Finally, test function by asking the patient to do up a shirt button, hold an object such as a key or a pen, etc.

If when the fingers are extended (from a grip) one of the fingers stays flexed, consider Dupuytren's or trigger finger. Dupuytren's disease usually affects the ring and little fingers (see section on Dupuytren's disease). Ask the patient if they can straighten the finger themselves. In Dupuytren's disease they will tell you they cannot. If they can straighten it (usually with a snap), this is likely to be a trigger finger.

Trigger finger is usually caused by thickening of the fibrous tendon sheath, perhaps due to repetitive trauma. Feel along the palm (volar) aspect of the hand (just distal to the MCPJs). In a trigger finger you may feel a thickening of the sheath which rolls under your finger as the patient flexes and extends their finger. This also happens to be the location for a small ganglion, sometimes referred to as a pearl ganglion, because of its size and consistency, and is worth a mention as it is a differential diagnosis.

FRACTURE CLASSIFICATION AND MANAGEMENT

A fracture is a break in the continuity of a bone. It should be thought of as a soft tissue injury around a broken bone, since often more problems can arise from the soft tissue damage than from the fracture itself.

Fractures can be open or closed, intra- or extra-articular, and displaced or undisplaced. In closed fractures the skin remains intact. Open fractures (which used to be called "compound") are fractures where the surface wound communicates with the fracture and there is thus potential for contamination through the wound. (Note that the wound does not necessarily have to be to the skin and may be an internal body surface, such as the rectum.) You cannot tell from an X-ray whether a fracture is open or closed.

Types of Fracture

Types of fracture pattern include transverse, oblique, spiral, multifragmentary (i.e. more than two fragments, and used to be called comminuted), avulsion (a bony fragment being torn off by a tendon or ligament), compression (or crush, which occurs when cancellous bone is crumpled, such as in the vertebral bodies, especially in the presence of osteoporosis) and stress fractures (these occur after repeated stresses that cause the bone to fatigue, often seen in the lower limbs of athletes) (Figure 15.1). Two other types you need to know about are greenstick and pathological fractures.

Greenstick fractures are seen in children, whose bones are softer and more pliable and tend to bend rather than break. The cortex on one side tends to buckle (imagine bending a young green twig — hence the name "greenstick").

Pathological fractures are fractures occurring in a bone that has already been weakened by disease, and may occur with normal physiological stresses. There are many causes, including generalised bone diseases or metastatic deposits in the bone. One could think of pathological fractures as being of two types: one where a fracture occurs in a patient with generalised bone disease, such as a crushed vertebra or a fractured neck of femur in an osteoporotic lady; the other type occurs in patients with normal bone structure, but the fracture is in a localised area of abnormal bone, such as through a metastatic deposit. Osteoporosis is the commonest cause of pathological fracture, especially in the spine and femoral neck. Although strictly speaking osteoporotic fractures are pathological, in practice we do not tend to refer to them as being pathological, otherwise most of the fractures in the geriatric age group

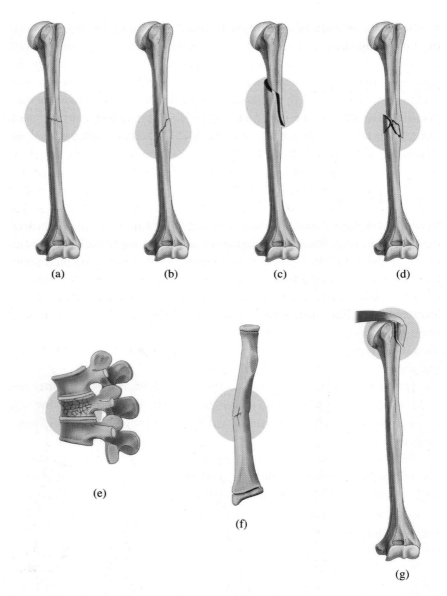

Figure 15.1.   Types of fracture: (a) transverse, (b) oblique, (c) spiral, (d) comminuted, (e) crush, (f) greenstick, (g) avulsion.

would be "pathological". The term is usually reserved for those involving malignancies.

Displacement of Fractures

When a bone breaks, the fragments often displace due to the force of the injury and also due to gravity and the pull of muscles attached to the fragments. There are many terms used to describe displacement, such as "impaction", "angulation", "translation", "opposition" and "rotation" (Figure 15.2). Impaction implies that the fragments are driven into one another, causing shortening. Angulation (or malalignment) means that one fragment is angulated in relation to the other, which if left alone may lead to deformity of the limb. Angulation is described in degrees whereas translation is measured as a percentage. Whenever describing displacement, always refer to the distal fragment relative to the proximal fragment.

Dislocation is complete loss of congruity between the articulating surfaces of a joint. The term implies disruption to the capsule and soft tissues

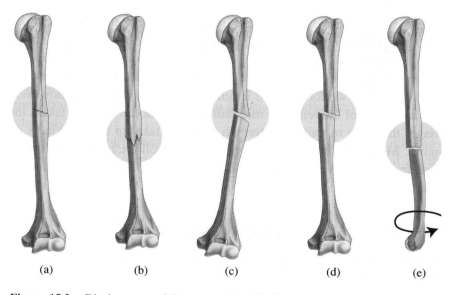

(a)	(b)	(c)	(d)	(e)

Figure 15.2. Displacement of fractures: (a) undisplaced, (b) impacted, (c) angulated (25°), (d) lateral displacement (i.e. 50% opposed or 50% translated), (e) rotation.

- *Continuous traction.* This is either skin or skeletal traction and can be maintained for several weeks. In adults it does not tend to be used much nowadays, due to the problems of prolonged bed rest and also for social and economic reasons. One common example of traction used nowadays is the collar and cuff for certain shoulder fractures, where the weight of the arm is used as the force of distraction. Gallows traction, another example, is used to treat children (less than two years old) with femoral fractures.

- *An external fixator (ex-fix).* The bony fragments are held in position by pins inserted through the skin and into the bone. The pins are then joined together with some external mechanical support. This method is especially useful in the management of open fractures where internal fixation with permanent metalwork may in some cases be inadvisable due to the higher risk of infection. Any patient with an ex-fix needs to be educated about pin site hygiene as it is not uncommon for the pin sites to become infected. In the case of deep infection the pins have to be removed.

- *Internal fixation.* Pins, plates, screws or large intramedullary nails are used to hold the bony fragments in position. They are usually left in permanently, although they can be removed if necessary once the fracture has united. Sometimes a bone graft (see section on non-union) is used to aid fracture healing, especially if there are large areas of bone loss. Internal fixation is used when the reduction needs to be as near perfect as possible (such as when a joint surface is involved), and also in the management of certain fractures to aid early mobility of the patient (e.g. hip fractures) or where it will not be possible to maintain an acceptable position by splintage or traction alone (very unstable fractures). One of the current buzzwords is "locking plates". Locking plates were introduced in the 1990s and are where the screw heads are threaded and, when tightened, lock into threads in the plate. They therefore provide a stable construct and act as a type of internal external fixator. Many surgeons now use them in preference to normal plates and screws, especially in soft osteoporotic bone, although full details on this are perhaps beyond the scope of this book and suffice for you to have heard of them.

Rehabilitation

Just because one part of the body is injured does not mean that the patient has to stay in bed and rest. The remaining limbs should be mobilised to avoid other complications. It is often quoted that immobility leads to a reduction in muscle mass of approximately 50% within two weeks.

The rehabilitation of the affected part really depends on the type of fracture. For example, after a hip operation it is important to get the patient up and mobilised as soon as possible. The physiotherapists are involved early and help with exercises and mobility. Rehabilitation involves restoring not only the injured part, but also the patient as a whole. This means an occupational therapist should help with various splints, mobility aids and home modifications, and the social services should be involved to increase resources such as home helps and meals on wheels.

Listed earlier are all of the options for the management of fractures; you will, however, find that two surgeons at different hospitals may differ markedly in the way they treat the same fracture. This is because the decision on how a fracture should be treated is not straightforward and depends on many factors, including the following:

- The nature of the accident and the complexity of the fracture
- The condition of the skin and soft tissues
- Any associated injuries
- The age, general health and personality of the patient
- The facilities available
- The skill of the surgeon

COMPLICATIONS OF FRACTURES

General Complications

Complications of Any Tissue Damage

- Haemorrhage and shock
- Fat embolism and respiratory distress syndrome
- Infection
- Muscle damage and rhabdomyolysis

Examples of nerve palsies include axillary nerve palsy (dislocation of the shoulder); radial nerve palsy (fracture of the shaft of the humerus); ulnar nerve palsy (elbow dislocation); sciatic nerve palsy (dislocated hip); and common peroneal nerve palsy (fracture of the neck of the fibula or knee dislocation). Nerve palsies are usually reversible, although it can sometimes take months before the function returns to normal.

Problems with Union

Delayed Union vs. Non-union

There is no exact time that a fracture should take to heal, but some fractures take longer than would be expected (for a person of that age), and this is called delayed union. If the bone fails to unite, then the fracture eventually goes on to a state of non-union. There is no exact distinction in terms of the time when you should call it delayed as opposed to non-union; however, if the bone has failed to unite after several months, it is unlikely to heal without intervention and is described as non-union. The cause of delayed union and non-union is unknown but, undoubtedly, poor blood supply, excessive shearing forces between the fragments, infection, interposition of tissue between the fragments could all contribute.

There are two types of non-union: hypertrophic and atrophic. Each has a characteristic X-ray appearance. Usually the bone ends look rounded (like elephant feet) and appear dense and sclerotic, and this is called hypertrophic non-union. In some cases a false joint may form (pseudoarthrosis) between the two ends. In these cases there is plenty of new bone formation but for some reason the two ends do not unite (perhaps because of movement or interposed tissues). Less commonly, the bone can look osteopenic, and it is then called atrophic non-union, which is probably due to inadequate blood supply.

In the case of a non-union the patient may require an operation such as ORIF and/or bone grafting to help the fracture unite (see section on bone grafting).

Factors Employed to Encourage Bone Healing

The most important thing to get a bone to heal is stability. Another tool is bone grafting. Bone graft has traditionally been taken from the patient's iliac crest. This is a painful procedure and often the wound over the donor site causes greater morbidity to the patient than the main operative site. This type of bone graft has no structural integrity and only acts as a framework on which new bone grows (i.e. a graft extender).

There are now a number of commercially available bone graft substitutes with the intention of reducing donor site morbidity and improving the chances of bony union. These include demineralised bone matrix, bone morphogenetic proteins (e.g. BMP-2 or OP-1) and bone graft substitutes. This is a growing field of orthopaedics. However, as with all advances, many surgeons argue that longer-term results of clinical trials are needed before they are prepared to change their practice.

Malunion

This is where the fracture has healed in an imperfect position, either shortened, angulated or rotated. It may cause an unsightly appearance despite good function, or it may look fine but functionally have a poor result (especially if a joint is involved). Worse still, it may be both.

Avascular Necrosis (AVN) (see p. 340)

Avascular necrosis is the death of part of a bone due to a deficient blood supply. Common sites for this to occur include the head of the femur, the scaphoid and the talus after fractures or dislocations where the blood supply is disrupted. The affected bones become soft and deformed, causing pain, stiffness and osteoarthritis. X-ray changes include sclerosis of the affected bone, which may appear distorted in shape; however, symptoms usually appear before any radiological changes.

Complex Regional Pain Syndrome (CRPS) Type I (Old Names: Reflex Sympathetic Dystrophy or Sudeck's Atrophy)

This is a collection of symptoms, including persistent pain, swelling, redness and sweating, thought to be due to an abnormal sympathetic response to injury (the nerves themselves are thought to be intact). There is a CRPS Type II which has similar symptoms but there is thought to be an underlying nerve injury. CRPS Type I is usually not noticed until the plaster has been removed, several weeks after the injury. For example, a small proportion of patients following a Colles' fracture have swelling of the hands and fingers, the skin is warm, pink and glazed in appearance, movement is decreased, and the wrist and hand are painful to touch. It can also be seen in the lower limb. Patients should be encouraged to move the affected limb as immobilisation can often make CRPS worse. Although the condition is usually self-limiting, some patients find it disabling and need the care of anaesthetic pain specialists. Guanethidine nerve blocks and sympathectomy can help in some cases.

Myositis Ossificans (Posttraumatic Ossification)

This is a condition where calcification forms in soft tissues following injury or surgery. It causes restricted, painful movement. The commonest site for this is the elbow region. The exact cause is unknown but is thought to be due to calcification and then ossification of blood that collected during the trauma. The affected area may be excised surgically at a later date if necessary.

Growth Disturbance

X-rays in children are difficult to interpret, as the growth plate is often confused for a fracture. If there is damage to the growth plate (physis — see section on bone tumours for an explanation on the physis), abnormal growth may result. Injuries at the epiphyseal end of long bones of children can be categorised according to the Salter–Harris classification into five types (Figure 15.4). The results of these injuries depend on the injury pattern and the management at the time of injury. Type I injuries tend to do well, whereas Type V injuries often do badly.

If a fracture goes through the epiphyseal plate (e.g. Salter–Harris I), provided good reduction is achieved there may be normal growth. Small

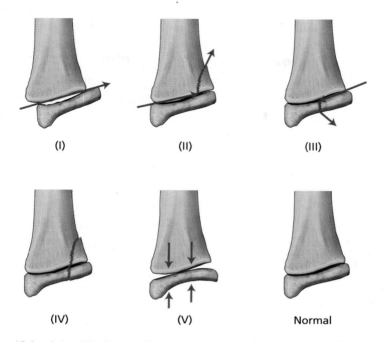

(I)   (II)   (III)

(IV)   (V)   Normal

Figure 15.4. Salter–Harris classification of epiphyseal injuries. Note the red lines indicate the site of the fracture injury. In Type I the injury goes through the growth plate leaving the bones intact. In Type II (the commonest type) the fracture exits through the metaphysical bone. In Type V the physis is crushed.

amounts of displacement are often acceptable in children's fractures, since they tend to remodel as the child grows (especially in the plane of movement). The worst fractures are the ones where a growth plate injury, such as a crush (e.g. Salter–Harris V), is missed at the time of the injury and is not picked up until growth is distorted. Many fractures in children can be treated by manipulation under anaesthetic and then immobilisation in plaster. The exceptions to this are intra-articular epiphyseal injuries, which require anatomical reduction and are usually treated by ORIF.

FRACTURES YOU SHOULD KNOW SOMETHING ABOUT

Fractures of the Neck of the Femur

These are often referred to as fractures of the proximal femur. They occur mainly in elderly females, usually with osteoporotic bone, and are therefore by definition pathological fractures. There is usually a history of a fall with the patient being unable to get up afterwards (in some cases the fracture may occur spontaneously and precede the fall).

These fractures have a high mortality (up to 40% at one year) no matter what treatment is performed in the initial period. The exact reason for this high mortality is unclear (even if you take into account the age and coexisting medical problems) and is studied all the time.

The normal finding on examination is to see the leg lying externally rotated and shortened. The iliopsoas muscle attaches to the lesser trochanter of the femur. If the fracture is proximal to this attachment, then the pull of this muscle causes the affected limb to lie shortened and externally rotated. This explains the classic clinical appearance of the limb in a fractured neck of femur. All movements may be painful and they usually cannot bear weight.

When clerking the patient you should pay particular attention to four factors:

- Premorbid mobility
- Mini-mental test score
- Premorbid independence
- Comorbidity

When documenting the patient's social circumstances, you should focus on what their mobility had been like prior to the fall. Were they walking independently or did they need a stick or frame? Do they live alone, in a warden-controlled flat or in a nursing home? How many floors and stairs does their house have and who does the shopping, cleaning and cooking? You should also document the patient's mini-mental test score. In general the prognosis is better if the patient was cognitively intact, mobile and independent previously. This will also give you a guide as to what they will be likely to achieve afterwards.

If the patient has a history of a fall and clinical findings support the diagnosis of a fractured neck of the femur but the X-rays appear normal, then a magnetic resonance imaging (MRI) might need to be requested.

Fractured necks of femurs are classified as intra- or extracapsular, depending on whether the fracture is proximal or distal to the capsular insertion (which is along the intertrochanteric line) (Figure 15.5).

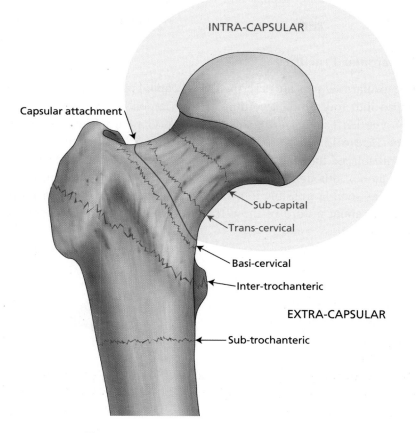

Capsular attachment

INTRA-CAPSULAR

Sub-capital

Trans-cervical

Basi-cervical

Inter-trochanteric

EXTRA-CAPSULAR

Sub-trochanteric

Figure 15.5.   Types of fractured neck of the femur.

The main blood supply to the head of the femur comes from vessels that travel under the capsule and along the neck (a small supply is also derived from nutrient vessels in the shaft and from a vessel that travels in the ligamentum teres). Therefore, if a fracture is intracapsular, the blood supply to the head is often compromised, especially if displaced. It is impossible to tell which fractures will go on to develop avascular necrosis, but logic tells you that the more displaced the head is, the more likely the vessels will have been torn and hence the higher the chance of avascular necrosis. Extracapsular fractures, on the other hand, usually have an intact blood supply and therefore a lower risk of avascular necrosis.

Intracapsular Fractures

Intracapsular fractures are described as subcapital or transcervical, and are grouped into four types according to the Garden classification (Garden I–IV). Garden I and II are undisplaced and Garden III and IV are displaced (Figure 15.6).

Undisplaced intracapsular fractures are often impacted and will unite if left alone, although the aim nowadays is usually to mobilise such patients as soon as possible to avoid the complications of prolonged bed rest. Also, about a third of these fractures will go on to displace if not

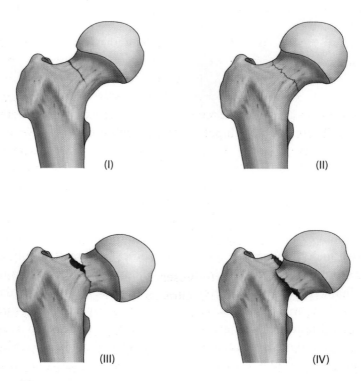

(I)   (II)

(III)   (IV)

Figure 15.6.   The Garden classification of intracapsular fractures.

fixed. In most cases, therefore, the fracture is stabilised at operation, usually by the insertion of parallel screws through the neck and into the head to hold it in position.

Displaced intracapsular fractures will not usually unite without reduction (Figure 15.7a). Because of the disrupted blood supply to the head of the femur, many of such patients go on to develop avascular necrosis. Now, following the general principles of fracture management, it would be perfectly reasonable to treat such fractures by reducing the fracture and holding it in position with screws. However, if you follow up patients in whom the fracture is reduced and held with screws, over the next few months many of them will still have pain and require a second operation (due to AVN of the femoral head). For this reason, many surgeons would recommend excising the femoral head and replacing it with a prosthesis (hemiarthroplasty, or half a hip replacement) at the initial operation. In young patients (less than 65) they might even recommend a total hip replacement.

There are many types of hemiarthroplasty available. The Thompson and Austin Moore prostheses have been around for decades. With hemiarthroplasties the false head is large and articulates directly with the patient's acetabulum. The Austin Moore is an example of an uncemented prosthesis (Figure 15.7b), the Thompson or JRI are examples of cemented prostheses. There are also bipolar hemiarthoplasties that have a small head which fits inside a larger head that sits in the acetabulum (Figure 15.7c). Theoretically there is reduced wear on the acetabulum due to sharing of the articulation between the small head and the large head and between the large head and the patient's acetabulum.

In the young patient (aged less than 65) you need to consider the long-term outcome. The disruption to the blood supply is dependent on the severity of the initial trauma, but early reduction may prevent subsequent AVN. Ideally, you want to preserve the patient's own joint for as long as possible. Therefore, all intracapsular fractures in the young should be booked for theatre as an emergency and undergo reduction and have internal fixation (usually with screws). Young patients should be followed up in the outpatient clinic for at least two years and if they develop AVN, could be considered for a total hip replacement at a later date.

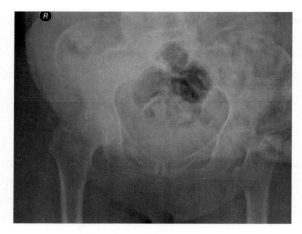

(a)

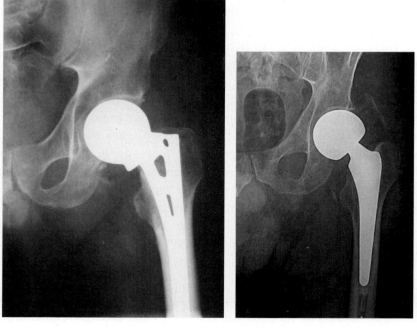

(b)   (c)

Figure 15.7.   (a) Displaced intracapsular fractured neck of the femur (left); (b) Austin Moore (uncemented) hemiarthroplasty (left); (c) bipolar hemiarthroplasty (note the stem is cemented).

Extracapsular Fractures

Extracapsular fractures can be described as basicervical, intertrochanteric or subtrochanteric, depending on the relationship to the trochanters (Figure 15.8a).

Extracapsular fractures do not carry the same risk of avascular necrosis and if minimally displaced, could be managed non-operatively. Again, however, most orthopaedic surgeons advocate early mobilisation. As it is not possible to mobilise easily if the hip is fractured and unstable, we tend to fix these fractures. Fixing these fractures will also help to reduce the amount of pain.

The standard operation nowadays for these fractures is the insertion of a dynamic hip screw (DHS) (Figure 15.8b). In this procedure the patient is placed on a special "fracture" table and the foot is placed into a traction boot. A closed reduction is performed (whereby traction is applied to the leg, under image intensifier control, to reduce the fracture). An incision is made over the greater trochanter and a screw is inserted into the femoral head under image intensifier control. A plate attaches to the DHS and rests along the shaft of the femur, to which it is fixed by screws. The angle between the plate and the screw is 135°, which is the usual angle between the neck and the shaft in most people (note: different angles are available to cover anatomical variants).

These fractures have a natural tendency to collapse and so the screw can slide along the plate to accommodate this. The screw can slide but cannot rotate. The sliding movement of the screw on the plate explains why the hip screw is "dynamic". This type of collapse is a good thing as it leads to a more stable construct.

In summary, the management of a patient with a hip fracture involves the following:

- Obtain a good history and social status for the patient.
- Insert a cannulae and send off bloods for urea and electrolytes (U&E), full blood count (FBC) and a group and save.
- If necessary, correct any medical problems (the patients are usually dehydrated and require fluid resuscitation), optimising them for theatre.

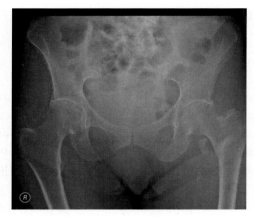

(a)

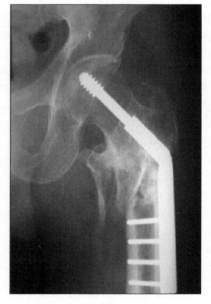

(b)

Figure 15.8.   (a) Extracapsular fractured neck of the femur (left) — note this is a four-part fracture as the lesser and greater trochanters are fractured, as well as a fracture line extending across the intertrochanteric region; (b) dynamic hip screw (DHS) fixation (left) — note the lesser trochanter remains displaced as it is not held by the metalwork and is under the strong pull of iliopsoas.

- Get an electrocardiogram (ECG) and a chest X-ray and an X-ray of the pelvis and affected limb.
- Mark the affected limb in preparation for theatre.
- Ensure the surgeon obtains informed consent.
- If the patient is in severe discomfort, skin traction can be applied to reduce the pain.

Extracapsular fractures are reduced and internally fixed (usually a DHS). Intracapsular fractures, if undisplaced, undergo fixation (screws), and if displaced, undergo a hemiarthroplasty. There is a saying commonly used by medical students that applies to intracapsular fractures classified by Garden: "One, two, screw, three, four Austin Moore." Whilst this catchy quip might help you to remember things, the Austin Moore prosthesis should be reserved only for the elderly who do not have too many mobility demands.

All young patients with intracapsular fractures should be given the best chance of survival of the femoral head and should be booked as an emergency to allow the fracture to be accurately reduced and internally fixed.

The management of these patients is multidisciplinary and should include a consultant orthogeriatrician on the team to manage their comorbidities, including secondary prevention for osteoporosis treatments. All efforts should be made to operate early (within 48 h of admission). DVT prophylaxis must be instituted as per the latest National Institute for Health and Clinical Excellence (NICE) guidelines (e.g. oral anticoagulants and thromboembolic deterrent or TED stockings/foot pumps, and early mobilisation).

Radius and Ulnar Shaft

Due to the anatomy, isolated fractures of the shafts of either of these bones are uncommon, and if they are seen one should always suspect an associated dislocation at either the proximal or the distal radioulnar joint. These fracture dislocations are known by their Italian eponyms and are common questions in exams, so they are worth remembering.

A fracture of the ulnar shaft with dislocation of the radial head is called a Monteggia fracture (the radial head should normally lie in front of the capitellum). A Galeazzi fracture is a fracture of the radial shaft with a dislocation of the distal (or inferior) radioulnar joint (Figure 15.9).

These fractures are unstable and are usually treated by ORIF in adults. In children the fracture is usually manipulated under anaesthetic (if displaced) and treated in an above-elbow plaster.

If a fracture of the forearm is being treated in plaster, then it should be left in the most stable position. Fractures of the proximal radius and ulna are said to be most stable in supination, distal fractures are said to be most stable in pronation, and fractures of the midshaft are said to be most stable in neutral. For example, a midshaft radial fracture is plastered with the hand in neutral (midpronation). The plaster is extended above the elbow to prevent any supination or pronation.

Fractures of the Distal Radius

Fractures of the distal radius are often associated with their eponymous names. In 1814 an Irishman called Abraham Colles described a deformity of the wrist, originally mistaken for a dislocated carpus. This was long

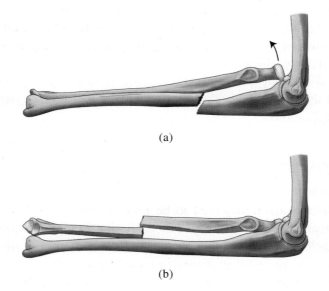

(a)

(b)

Figure 15.9.   Types of forearm fractures: (a) Monteggia fracture; (b) Galeazzi fracture.

before the invention of radiography and he showed that it was in fact not a dislocation but a fracture of the distal end of the radius. The deformity has been referred to as a "dinner-fork" deformity, because of how it looks.

These fractures can occur at any age after a fall onto an outstretched hand. However, they are most common in the elderly with osteoporosis. Colles' description was an extra-articular fracture of the distal radius within an inch and a half of the joint. The displacement of the distal fragment is dorsal with radial shift and impaction. There are many types of distal radial fracture, some of which can involve the joint and some of which involve the ulnar as well. You probably don't need to know all of the classifications for these fractures but the principles are that rotational injuries (often indicated by a fracture of the ulnar styloid) have more complex injury patterns and do worse than simple extra-articular fracture patterns.

On examination, as with any fracture, the neurovascular function should be documented. This is important because the median nerve and the radial artery lie close.

If the fracture is displaced, then treatment involves correction of the deformity and this is usually by manipulation. In cases where manipulation fails then the patient may require ORIF.

The reduction aims to improve two things: First, to restore the length (the articular surface of the distal radius should be more distal than the ulna), and second, to correct the angulation to allow for optimum function and minimal deformity.

Reduction, as always, is achieved by distraction in the direction opposite to the forces which caused it in the first place. In this case the wrist is left in a neutral or slightly flexed position with some ulnar deviation. A Colles plaster is applied from the elbow to just short of the metacarpophalangeal joints, leaving them free to move. The plaster encompasses the thumb metacarpal, again leaving the thumb metacarpophalangeal joint free to move.

If the fracture is suspected to be rotationally unstable, in an ideal world, the plaster should be above-elbow to prevent supination and pronation. Sadly, however, the risk of shoulder and elbow stiffness is so great that we tend to leave the plaster below-elbow, especially in the elderly. In children who will move things as soon as they can, an above-elbow plaster is usually applied from the start.

normal, the plaster can be removed and the patient discharged. If the X-ray is still normal but the patient is still tender, then the plaster should really be replaced for a further two weeks. In difficult cases, an MRI scan is helpful in making the diagnosis.

The main concern with this fracture is the risk of avascular necrosis. The blood supply to the scaphoid is via small vessels that enter the bone distally and hence the proximal fragment is at risk of becoming avascular (especially if displaced), leaving the patient with pain and stiffness in the wrist.

Scaphoid fractures require a plaster for at least six weeks, after which time the wrist is reassessed by X-rays and clinical examination. If a complication such as delayed union or non-union occurs, then either the arm can be placed in a plaster for a further six weeks or ORIF and bone grafting may be considered. ORIF usually involves a screw across the fracture site with or without bone grafting. Some surgeons do this percutaneously.

Supracondylar Fractures of the Humerus

These injuries are most common in children, usually after a fall onto an outstretched hand. The elbow is very swollen and is held in a semi-flexed position. The distal fragment usually displaces backwards and the sharp edge of the proximal humerus may compress or injure the brachial artery which lies just in front of it (Figure 15.10).

The key to management is first to ensure no neurovascular damage occurs and second to restore the anatomy to prevent long-term malunion.

If the fracture is angulated with a clinical deformity then the child needs to be admitted and have the fracture manipulated under anaesthesia with image intensifier control. If there is any evidence of a neurovascular deficit then this needs to be immediate. Once satisfactory reduction is obtained, the position needs to be held and this is usually achieved by placing a few short K-wires across the fracture (being careful to protect the ulnar nerve). Then a collar and cuff or a back slab is applied again with the arm fully flexed. If the radial pulse is weak or not present then the arm will need to be straightened a little until it returns. If the radial pulse is not present or damage to the brachial artery is suspected, an on-table angiogram and or exploration needs to take place.

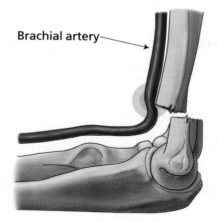

Brachial artery

Figure 15.10.   Supracondylar fracture of the humerus.

If the fracture is non-displaced then the treatment is to flex the arm fully (checking the radial pulse). The sling provided by the triceps insertion, when the arm is fully flexed, helps to stabilise the fragments. One could also apply a back slab if necessary for a few days just to prevent the arm from being knocked. The immobilisation is usually about two weeks in a young child.

Any supracondylar fracture is at risk of compartment syndrome, and so the child needs to be observed very carefully over the first 24 h. Pain on passive extension (stretching the flexor compartment) of the fingers is the earliest warning sign of compartment syndrome. The elbow should be extended slightly to see if this restores the circulation, but if this fails surgical intervention may be needed, otherwise Volkmann's ischaemic contracture can result. This is where the forearm muscles become fibrosed and shortened, leading to a "claw-hand" deformity.

If a supracondylar fracture is missed or the reduction is inadequate, deformity can result. Angular deformities in the coronal plane do not remodel and can result in loss of the carrying angle and cubitus varus. If there is cubitus varus, internal rotation and extension of a healed supracondylar fracture, this is referred to as a "gunstock deformity", because of the unsightly appearance. Despite the fact that function is usually quite good, these deformities should not really be seen these days with appropriate orthopaedic management.

Dislocated Shoulder

Because the shoulder is the most mobile of all the joints, its stability is sacrificed, especially inferiorly where the rotator cuff is deficient. In addition, in some patients there is underlying laxity of ligaments.

Almost all cases of dislocation of the shoulder are anterior dislocations (95%). Dislocation is usually caused by direct trauma or falling onto the hand where the humerus is driven forwards, tearing the capsule of the joint. Often the glenoid labrum is pulled off anteriorly, and this is called a Bankart lesion. If the humeral head impacts against the relatively hard anterior glenoid, a defect can occur on the superior surface of the humeral head, called a Hill–Sachs lesion. This occurs in 35–40% of anterior dislocations. A Hill–Sachs lesion may destabilise the glenohumeral joint and predispose to further dislocation.

The patient presents in severe pain and is reluctant to undergo any examination of the shoulder. The normal curved contour of the shoulder may be lost and may appear square. The arm is supported by the opposite hand. It is vital that you examine for any distal neurovascular deficit, especially of the axillary nerve, which can be damaged during the dislocation. The axillary nerve supplies a small egg-shaped patch of skin over the insertion of the deltoid and should be tested and findings documented both before and after reduction (the axillary nerve also supplies the deltoid but clearly the muscle is difficult to assess whilst the shoulder is dislocated).

X-rays should be taken from AP and transscapular views (in the line of the body of the scapula) to see in which direction the humeral head has gone in relation to the glenoid, i.e. anterior or posterior.

Reduction is usually performed under sedation in the casualty department. One method has the patient in the supine position with the arm abducted, and an assistant applying countertraction to the body (maybe with a towel held around the patient's chest under the axilla). The head can be guided gently back into the socket.

An alternative is to have the patient prone with the arm hanging attached to some weights to apply traction. Kocher's method is written about in most A&E textbooks but research has shown that whilst this method is effective at reducing shoulders, the reduction method also often slices off the articular cartilage on the rim of the glenoid and so the author does not recommend this manoeuvre and prefers gentler traction alone.

If closed reduction methods fail, then reduction is usually easy to achieve with some muscle relaxant in theatre.

The arm can then be rested in a sling for a few days, after which physiotherapy rehabilitation can begin. The patient is advised against positions that can increase the likelihood of dislocation, namely abduction and external rotation such as throwing a baseball or when swinging back to serve in tennis.

Recurrent Instability

After an initial dislocation, the shoulder may return to functional stability or it may fall victim to recurrent glenohumeral instability. The older a patient is at the time of initial injury the lower the chances are for developing recurrent instability. Patients under the age of 20 with traumatic dislocations have a substantially higher rate of recurrence (greater than 90%).

While intermediate forms of recurrent instability do occur, the great majority of recurrently unstable shoulders may be thought of as being either atraumatic or traumatic in origin.

Two terms are described which you may find useful to understand shoulder instability. These are TUBS and AMBRI.

Traumatic Unilateral Dislocations with a Bankart lesion often require Surgery (TUBS). Most dislocations are traumatic and patients presenting with TUBS are usually between the ages of 15 and 30. Surgery usually involves a Bankart repair whereby the glenoid labrum is reattached to the glenoid, usually by using bone anchors and sutures.

Atraumatic instability is instability that arises without the type of trauma necessary to tear the stabilising soft tissues and is often bilateral. It is called AMBRI because this stands for Atraumatic Multidirectional Bilateral shoulder dislocation (or subluxation) and is best treated by Rehabilitation but occasionally should be considered for an Inferior capsular shift.

Management of shoulder instability requires careful diagnosis based on the history, examination and imaging. Operating on an AMBRI without careful diagnosis beforehand may lead to poor results.

Posterior Dislocation

Posterior dislocation of the shoulder is easily overlooked (and occasionally you will see a patient who sustained a posterior dislocation several days or weeks prior that had been missed). It is caused by direct trauma (and is seen in epileptics). The AP X-ray may give the impression of the humeral head sitting in the glenoid (hence it is missed), although it may appear rounded — the so-called "light bulb" sign (due to internal rotation, and hence the greater tuberosity is not seen). Reduction is best performed by a specialist.

Inferior Dislocation

This is the least likely form of shoulder dislocation but worth mentioning due to the unusual presentation. This type of dislocation is also known as luxatio erecta because the arm is held permanently upwards (the humeral head is sitting under the glenoid and the arm is hyperabducted). Inferior dislocations are associated with a high complication rate and can result in vascular, neurological or tendon injuries. Reduction of such injuries should be performed by an expert.

Femoral and Tibial Fractures

In these injuries, resuscitate the patient and deal with life-threatening injuries first. Blood loss can be great, so cross-match two units in tibial fractures and four units in femoral fractures. A traction splint can be applied for femoral fractures, and a padded board or long leg splint can be used for tibial fractures. Both injuries are at risk of compartment syndrome. In the young most of these fractures are treated surgically. The state-of-the-art treatment for femoral or tibial fractures is to use an intramedullary nail (a long nail placed right down the centre from the top end to hold the fracture). There are alternative treatments, including a plate and screws or an external fixator. Each method has advantages and disadvantages (for example, the pins of an external fixator go through the muscles in the thigh, limiting rehabilitation), and for the sake of examinations you need to know that all are acceptable options. If the fracture is 'open'), management is different (see earlier section). Antibiotics are started, and the patient is taken to theatre for debridement and washout. The fracture is then assessed and stabilised.

There have been studies showing that patients who have their femoral fractures stabilised within 24 h do better in terms of respiratory complications (e.g. chest infection and adult respiratory distress syndrome (ARDS)) than patients who are left for longer before the operation. One of the main factors in this is that nursing care is made easier, allowing the patients to sit up once they have been fixed.

Knee Injuries

Knee injuries commonly affect sportsmen and questions on them are likely to come up in exams. Several structures can be damaged in the knee. The collateral ligaments get torn in valgus or varus strains. Twisting injuries can lead to meniscal tears or a rupture of the anterior cruciate ligament and there is a triad that can follow a severe rotational injury where the anterior cruciate, the medial meniscus and the medial collateral ligament are all torn ("the unhappy triad of O'Donoghue").

History

The time of presentation will dictate the types of questions you should ask in your history. For example, if assessment is shortly after the injury, the only questions you can ask are related to the mechanism of injury and previous injuries to this knee.

If presentation is delayed, for example until the next day or longer, then you must ask whether the knee swelled up immediately or overnight. If the knee swelled immediately, this points to a haemarthrosis, which often occurs with fractures or torn cruciates. Overnight swelling indicates an effusion, which may in turn imply a meniscal tear or another ligamentous injury.

If the patient presents some time after the injury, then an accurate history invariably points to the diagnosis. Symptoms that you should ask about include the four cardinal knee symptoms, namely, pain, locking, swelling and giving way. Locking means that the patient cannot fully extend the knee because of a mechanical obstruction, such as a meniscal tear. Giving way is usually a sign of instability, such as that which can follow a torn ACL, but may occur because of pain. A history of locking, together with the finding of an effusion and joint line tenderness, usually indicates a meniscal tear.

Management

If a patient presents immediately after the injury, with an acutely swollen knee, full examination is often difficult. You will note the extent of the swelling and which areas are tender as well as the range of movement. Testing for menisci or cruciate damage when the knee is acutely swollen can be quite difficult. If the mechanism of injury dictates, then an X-ray can be taken to ensure there are no fractures. A lateral X-ray might reveal a fluid level indicating a lipohaemarthrosis (mixture of fat and blood in a joint cavity). Even in the absence of an obvious fracture, this should set off alarm bells as it could indicate a torn ACL or an osteochondral injury.

The management of an acutely swollen knee (without fractures) is usually Rest, Ice packs, Compression or splintage, and Elevation (RICE). After a few days, once the swelling has subsided, the knee can be re-examined for meniscal, ligamentous or chondral damage.

If a meniscal tear or torn cruciate is suspected, then an MRI scan can be performed to confirm the diagnosis. Some surgeons will take a look into the knee in the absence of an MRI if they are certain of the diagnosis.

An arthroscopy means the knee is looked into with a camera. It is imperative that the knee is re-examined under anaesthesia before the arthroscope is inserted into the knee. With the patient asleep and the muscle tone reduced, it is far easier to assess the stability.

The arthroscope is inserted through an incision, just lateral to the patellar tendon, into the lateral compartment of the knee. A second incision is made into the medial compartment where a probe is inserted. This way the surgeon has the ability to look, feel, touch and pull various structures as part of the examination.

The three joint compartments are inspected — the patellofemoral joint and the medial and lateral compartments. If a meniscal tear is seen it can be trimmed using various instruments and shavers. There are many types of meniscal tears, an example being a "bucket-handle" tear, where the "bucket handle" can flip in and out of the joint space, causing locking.

In years gone by, surgeons used to remove torn menisci but we now know that this predisposes to osteoarthritis and so the menisci must be preserved as much as possible. Only the outer third of the meniscus has a blood supply and tears of this region are usually repaired using sutures or newer devices. Tears in the inner third have to be trimmed because they are not repairable. When a tear is in the junction of the middle to outer third (referred to as the white-red zone), a difficult decision is made and depending on the age of the patient, the surgeon may attempt a repair.

Aside from the menisci, the other things inspected in an arthroscopy include the articular surfaces, the cruciate ligaments and the various soft tissue pouches, such as the lateral gutter, medial gutter and suprapatellar pouch, in order to look for loose bodies. The joint is irrigated with several litres of normal saline during an arthroscopy and so infection is rare.

Postoperatively, early mobilisation is encouraged, if necessary with the use of crutches until the pain subsides.

Management of a Ruptured Anterior Cruciate Ligament

A torn anterior cruciate ligament can lead to instability especially during twisting and cutting movements that are common in sports. The treatment after rupture of the ACL may be operative or conservative. In both cases, the goal is to reach the best functional level for the patient without risking new injuries or degenerative changes in the knee.

Rehabilitation is an important part of the treatment. By strengthening up the quads and hamstrings and starting proprioceptive exercises it is possible to stabilise the knee without surgery in about a third of cases.

Operative repair involves the use of a tendon (allograft or autograft) or an artificial graft. The results of artificial grafts have so far been poor and nowadays the gold standard involves the use of either the middle third of the patellar tendon or the hamstring tendon (autografts). Allografts are tendons from cadavers and tend to be reserved for revisions or cases where multiple tendons need replacing. The tendon is rerouted through the knee in the same location as the old torn ACL and held using a screw.

In the US over 50,000 ACL reconstructions take place each year and in the UK about 5000. Long-term results depend on what assessment criteria you are using. Return to high level of athletic activity has been an indicator of treatment success and indeed if this is the outcome measure then ACL reconstruction is a very successful operation. If the outcome, however, is prevention of longer-term arthritis then we really don't know the answer. It is logical to assume that an unstable knee has a higher chance of developing osteoarthritis earlier than the same knee with an intact ACL. The confounding factors include other injuries, such as meniscal tears and damage to the articular surfaces at the time of injury. Also further injuries sustained subsequently will further confound the long-term results of any ACL repair. The definitive answer to the question "Will an ACL repair prevent me from getting osteoarthritis?" may never be found.

Current postoperative rehabilitation programmes encourage immediate range of motion. Commonly, the patients are allowed to return to light sporting activities such as running at 2–3 months after surgery and to contact sports, including cutting and jumping, after six months.

In less active patients a decision may be made to persist with non-operative management. Approximately a third of patients can develop sufficient stability without the need for surgery, mainly through muscular training and education. These patients are unlikely to be able to engage in activities that require very stable knees (for example, playing football or rugby) without risk of further damage.

In addition, the patient's occupation might influence the decision to operate, since a torn cruciate may not be as important in a person who works behind a desk as it is in a roofer who climbs up ladders.

Osteochondral Injuries

Articular cartilage (or hyaline cartilage — note that the word "hyaline" comes from the Greek for "glass") covers the articulating surfaces of bones within synovial joints and is crucial for their smooth articulation. It also serves to absorb shock by spreading the applied load to the bony supporting structures below. In most cases articular cartilage is able to carry out its task of strenuous load bearing for a lifetime.

However, cartilage is avascular, aneural and alymphatic and has a very low cell density and hence has limited intrinsic repair potential. If the surface becomes damaged and is left untreated, the initial damage will lead to further matrix disruption and the development of progressive degenerative arthritis. Sadly, up to a quarter of all severe ligament or capsular knee injuries that result in a haemarthrosis are associated with cartilage damage.

If left alone, partial-thickness lesions do not heal. However, if the lesion extends deep into the subchondral bone, so that bleeding occurs, some repair does ensue. The repair is due to the flow of stem cells from the marrow to the site. Surgical techniques were developed to replicate this, such as subchondral drilling, microfracture and abrasion arthroplasty; however, these methods have generally revealed the formation of fibrocartilage repair tissue, which lacks the same durability as hyaline cartilage and wears away quicker and thus does not represent a long-term solution. No one knows why fibrocartilage forms instead of hyaline cartilage.

Autologous chondrocytes have been used since the early 1990s. Autologous chondrocyte implantation (ACI) was pioneered by a Swedish group and in brief involves harvesting cartilage from the margins of the affected knee joint by arthroscopy. The cells are then cultured and expanded in numbers in a laboratory for about four weeks, after which they are transplanted back into the damaged area. The cells are held in position by a membrane of either artificial collagen or periosteum taken from the upper tibia. The membrane is sutured into position over the cartilage defect before injection of cells.

Newer techniques remove the need to suture a membrane over the defect. Two examples of such techniques include MACI® (matrix-associated chondrocyte implantation), where the chondrocytes are cultured directly onto the membrane, and this is then glued onto the defect during an arthroscopic procedure; and Chondron™, in which the cultured chondrocytes are mixed with the fibrin glue itself, and then placed directly into the defect in the absence of a collagen carrier.

Although short- to medium-term results of chondrocyte transplantation techniques have been promising, the longer-term outcome of this

painkillers they take. On examination movement is restricted, usually with accompanied crepitus, and in later stages of the disease there may be joint malalignment and fixed flexion deformities.

A top tip: When examining a patient, look at their hands. If you notice swellings in the fingers (Heberden's nodes at the DIPJs and Bouchard's nodes at the PIPJs) then this points to primary osteoarthritis as the diagnosis.

X-Ray Changes

OA has the following X-ray changes (Figure 15.11):

- Narrowing of the joint space (as the cartilage is worn away)
- Osteophytes — bits of bone overgrowth, usually near the edge of the joint
- Subchondral sclerosis

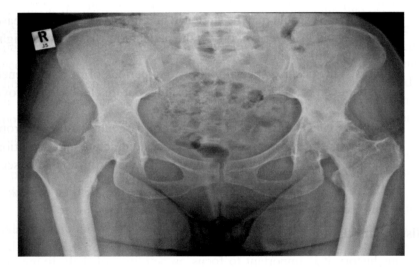

Figure 15.11. X-ray changes in osteoarthritis — the right hip has some osteoarthritic changes with narrowing of joint space, but nowhere near as severe as the left where the joint space is completely obliterated; there are bone cysts, subchondral sclerosis and osteophytes.

- Subchondral bone cysts
- There may be evidence of previous disorders, such as old fractures, rheumatoid or congenital defects
- Structural damage — bony destruction and deformity is a late sign

Management

In the early stages of the disease, treatment is conservative, using analgesics, weight loss, advice on altering load-bearing activities such as increasing periods of rest, using walking sticks or avoiding activities that exacerbate the condition. (In the younger patient this may mean giving up sports or changing job.) Physiotherapy to help increase the joint mobility and strengthen the muscles is often of great help. Injection of steroids and local anaesthetic into the joint space during acute flare-ups may be of some symptomatic benefit although it does nothing to treat the underlying arthritis. There is no strong evidence that intra-articular injections of hyaluronic acid-type substances are any better than placebo.

Patients often cope with their symptoms for many years. If, however, symptoms progress despite all of the above measures, then the following surgical options are available:

- *Arthroscopic washout.* The commonest site for this is the knee, and the severity of the disease is assessed directly and graded. The frayed cartilage can be trimmed and any loose bodies removed. Because the evidence to support arthroscopic washout is sparse, many primary care providers will no longer pay for such treatment on the NHS.
- *Osteotomy.* This means the bone is divided ("osteo" = bone and "tome" = cut), and sometimes a small area of the bone is removed to correct the deformity which is then fixed with plates and screws. Osteotomy can help relieve the pain but why it works is unknown. (It is thought that it may be due to adjustment of the weight-bearing surfaces and changes in blood flow to the bone.)
- *Arthrodesis.* This means the joint is fused and will therefore restrict mobility. It is mainly used as a last resort for joints where the loss of movement is not too disabling (for example, in the foot). For the hip and the knee, fusion is rarely performed nowadays as the results of

arthroplasty are so good. If infection is a high risk then arthrodesis might be preferred over arthroplasty.

- *Arthroplasty*. This can be replacement or excisional arthroplasty. The hip and the knee have received the most attention for replacement arthroplasty, although there are many other prostheses available for the shoulder, elbow and ankle, and almost any other joint. There is a now a National Joint Registry (NJR) in the UK that captures details of all patients having a hip, knee, shoulder or ankle replacement in the UK. The addition of other joints to the NJR is also being piloted. Joint replacement in the young remains a controversial subject, as the joint may only last 10–20 years and the results of revision surgery are not as good as those of primary surgery. Nowadays, however, some joint replacements are lasting longer and longer and are being used in younger age groups because the alternatives are nowhere near as good. In some joints, such as the interphalangeal joints of the toes, it is better to excise the arthritic joint, allowing a fibrous and pain-free joint to form in its place.

Total Hip Replacement (THR)

Total hip replacement was developed by Sir John Charnley in the 1960s and is now a very successful procedure for arthritis of the hip (with an expected survivorship of over ten years in 95% of cases). The worn acetabulum is replaced by a cup usually made of metal but lined by either high-density polyethylene, ceramic or metal. Into this cup articulates a femoral head which is made of either metal or ceramic. The components are either cemented in place using antibiotic-containing bone cement (methyl methacrylate) or are uncemented and coated or sintered to allow bone to grow into them (Figure 15.12).

For finals, you certainly do not have to know how to carry out a hip replacement, but for those of you who are interested, a brief overview is given here.

There are several operative approaches to the hip joint although the commonest are the anterolateral and posterior approaches. An incision is made over the greater trochanter and the fascia lata is divided. In the anterolateral approach, the abductors (gluteus medius and minimus) are

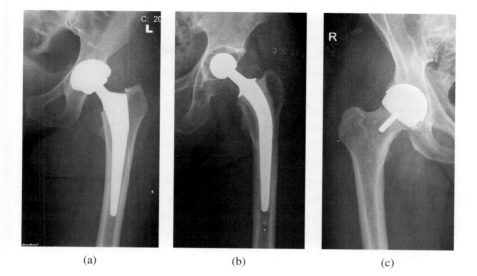

(a)   (b)   (c)

Figure 15.12.   Total hip replacement: (a) an uncemented hip replacement — both the acetabular and femoral components are uncemented; (b) a cemented acatabular and femoral component (note the white cement around the components); and (c) hip resurfacing.

lifted off the greater trochanter to gain access to the capsule of the joint. In the posterior approach, the short external rotators are divided and retracted to gain access to the capsule beneath (and to protect the sciatic nerve which lies close).

The capsule is incised. The head of the femur is dislocated and then the wear or damage to the acetabulum and femur can be assessed. The head of the femur is removed and the acetabulum is prepared using reamers to remove any cartilage and debris. The acetabular cup is inserted (cemented or uncemented). A hole is reamed down the femoral shaft and trials are initially used to assess the correct leg length and stability of the hip. Some prostheses nowadays are modular, meaning that different size neck lengths and different types of heads can be trialled for best fit. The head is relocated into the acetabulum and the function of the joint is tested to see if it is stable and the leg lengths are correct. The final components are then inserted to match the trials. The soft tissues are closed in layers. A reinfusion drain is often used to allow the lost blood to be reinfused postoperatively. The leg is placed in slight abduction using a triangular pillow, to maintain the joint in a good stable position.

Rehabilitation begins about a day or so after the operation, initially with leg exercises, and once the X-rays have been checked the patient is allowed to fully bear weight. The usual hospital stay is about 3–4 days although some patients go home sooner. Postoperative DVT prophylaxis is usually given for 28 days and can be subcutaneous low-molecular-weight heparin or an oral anticoagulant.

There are many hip replacements on the market (over 100) but only a smaller number have long-term published results. In the UK the NJR records data on all hip, knee and ankle replacements and data is now starting to inform practice.

For those with long-term results, the data suggests about 90% of THRs last over ten years. After about ten years, up to 10% can loosen and may need revision. However, the success rate of revision hips is not as good as the primary operation.

Main Complications of THR

- *Dislocation*. About 3% of primary THRs dislocate. Patients are advised of the positions that can be risky, including squatting or sitting on low chairs or movements that adduct the hip (i.e. sitting with crossed legs). There have been some studies suggesting that the posterior approach to the hip carries a higher rate of dislocation.
- *DVT*. Studies have shown that up to 50% of patients with THRs suffer a DVT and the risk is approximately halved with heparin prophylaxis. The risk of a PE is about 1–2% (although fatal PE is much lower). Nowadays, we tend to encourage early mobilisation together with TED stockings and possibly some form of chemical prophylaxis (oral or subcutaneous). The practice in most hospitals in the UK follows guidance from NICE, although there is a lack of convincing evidence in the literature.
- *Deep infection* (about 1–2%). This is disastrous and usually will require revision. A revision for infection can be single-stage or two-stage where the metalwork is removed in order to clear the infection

(a Girdlestone procedure) and traction is applied for several weeks before a definitive revision can be performed.

- *Nerve damage.* The sciatic nerve is just behind the hip joint and can be stretched during the procedure (especially posterior approaches) if care is not taken to protect it. This can lead to foot drop, which usually recovers but can take up to 18 months to do so. Also in the anterolateral approach the superior gluteal nerve can be injured, leading to weakness of the abductors and a Trendelenburg gait.
- *Leg length discrepancy.* Nowadays, with templating, patients should not be left with leg length discrepancies in primary hip replacements. Sometimes it is necessary to lengthen the components slightly, which tightens the soft tissues, to improve the stability of the hip but this leads to a slight leg length discrepancy. This usually can be addressed when the contralateral limb is operated on. Leg length discrepancy is usually not noticed if it is only a few millimeters, but patients have great problems with discrepancies of 1 cm or greater. A shoe raise can be tried.

Hip Resurfacing

Hip resurfacing where only the damaged surfaces are relined (in contrast to THR where the whole femoral head is resected) has always been an attractive concept. The theoretical advantages of hip resurfacings include reduced bone resection, closer restoration of normal anatomy and lower risk of dislocation.

Sir John Charnley, pioneer of THR, in fact carried out the first hip resurfacing in the 1950s using Teflon-on-Teflon bearings but unfortunately these Teflon bearings wore out quickly. The failure of materials plagued surgeons for the next 50 years but recently surgeons have developed new technologies that create perfect rounded bearing surfaces that allow very good clinical results and have been advocated for younger patients who want to restore as much bone stock as possible.

In these resurfacings the cap of the femoral head is replaced by a metal cover, as is the acetabulum, creating a metal-on-metal bearing surface (Figure 15.12c). Short- to medium-term results have been encouraging, although this is an emerging technology and long-term results are needed before it can become a mainstream procedure. There are also a few unanswered questions relating to this technology. One is the raised levels of cobalt and chromium ions in the blood after metal-on-metal surfaces are used. In the vast majority of patients with metal-metal hip resurfacing, there is an early rise in serum metal ions over the first 2–3 years but the levels then gradually diminish over time. The Medicines and Healthcare products Regulatory Agency (MHRA) recently issued a warning over the metal-on-metal issue, asking surgeons to be vigilant for problems in these patients, especially if they develop pain. In addition, one manufacturer withdrew their hip resurfacing product from the market due to a high revision rate, and hence there remains some uncertainty about the role for metal on metal hip replacements. Of course there is also a theoretical risk of carcinogenesis although no definitive data to support this risk has yet been published.

Total Knee Replacement (TKR)

Total knee replacement followed after THR. The success rate of this operation is almost as good as that of THR. We still tend to inform patients that the life of the joint replacement is about 10–20 years; however, some surgeons believe that a good knee replacement in a compliant patient can last a lifetime.

The joint is made of two metal prostheses with an intervening polyethylene articular disc between the distal femur and the tibial plateau. If only one compartment of the joint is damaged, this can be replaced by a unicompartmental prosthesis (mainly for the medial compartment). The whole joint is not replaced, just the articular surfaces (and hence joint resurfacing is perhaps a better name, in the same way as hip resurfacing). The materials used for the prostheses include titanium alloys, cobalt-chrome or stainless steel.

Again, for undergraduate exams you don't need to know the operative technique, but for those with an interest, an incision is made in front of the knee in the midline (about 20 cm long). The joint is accessed via the medial side of the patella as the patella is flipped back on itself (laterally) to get it out of the way. The distal femur and the tibial plateau are prepared by sawing off the irregular surfaces to allow the prostheses to fit on (using special jigs to ensure all the angles are correct). Trial prostheses are used to attain the correct sizes to allow for optimal function and stability of the joint. The prostheses are cemented into place and a polyethylene disc is inserted between the tibia and the femur, acting like the articular cartilage, ensuring that there is no contact between the metal parts. The anterior cruciate ligament is divided and the posterior cruciate is sometimes kept (PCL-retaining). If the patellar surface is worn, then it can also be resurfaced using a polyethylene button. The knee is washed out and the function is again tested, ensuring good flexion, patellar tracking and stability. Closure is again in layers, usually with a reinfusion drain to return lost blood to the patient (Figure 15.13).

Postoperatively, weight bearing and bending of the knee is begun the next day once the drain is removed. A check X-ray is taken on postoperative day 1. The patient is usually fit for discharge once the wound is looking good, the patient is safe at home, once extension and flexion of the knee are satisfactory and active straight leg raising is being achieved. The hospital stay is usually about 3–4 days. Postoperative DVT prophylaxis is usually given for 14 days and can be subcutaneous low–molecular-weight heparin or an oral anticoagulant.

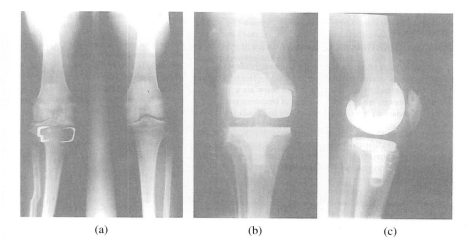

(a)   (b)   (c)

Figure 15.13. (a) Osteoarthritis of both knees — the medical compartment is more severely affected in both knees. Note that there are staples from an old right tibial osteotomy; (b) right total knee replacement (TKR). AP view; (c) lateral view (patellar surface has not been replaced).

Complications include DVT, which occurs in about 50–75% of TKRs (the incidence is halved if prophylaxis is used), although many are asymptomatic. The risk of pulmonary embolus is about 1% (although fatal PE is said to be <0.1%). The infection rate is about 2–3% and is a disaster because the success of revision knees is again much lower than that of the primary procedure.

RHEUMATOID ARTHRITIS (RA)

Rheumatoid arthritis is a large subject that usually comes up in the medical section of exams; however, there are many operative procedures that can be performed to help the patients and so below are a few lines on this subject. Answers are best related in terms of treatment goals, and for RA these include the following:

- *Prevention and treatment of the inflammatory synovitis*. Advice, exercises, joint protection and drugs such as the disease-modifying drugs — gold, penecillamine and immunosuppressants (methotrexate, pyrimidine synthesis inhibitors and anti-tumour necrosis factor (TNF) therapies).
- *Prevention of joint destruction and deformity*. Rest during acute exacerbations followed by rehabilitation and physiotherapy. RA patients are prone to tendon rupture, which may require operative repair.
- *Joint reconstruction*. Joint replacements have a place in RA patients. The hip, knee, shoulder, elbow and MCPJs are examples of joints which can be replaced in advanced destruction, deformity or instability. You must, however, treat the symptoms and not the X-ray appearances. Other operations that have a place are arthrodesis, osteotomy and synovectomy.

The X-ray changes of RA include soft tissue swelling, joint space narrowing and, later on, articular destruction and deformity.

AVASCULAR NECROSIS (AVN)

This often comes up in multiple choice questions. It is due to a disruption of the blood supply, either due to interruption of arterial inflow, such as after a fracture (covered earlier), or if venous outflow is blocked, as in infiltrative disorders that block the venous sinusoids (e.g. Gaucher's disease). The causes include the following:

- Fracture/dislocation
- Sickle cell disease (clumping of the red blood cells leads to diminished capillary flow. There is a tendency for the infarcted areas of bone to become infected with unusual organisms such as salmonella)
- Decompression sickness (caisson disease)
- Gaucher's disease (a rare familial disorder of lipid metabolism)
- Drug-induced (especially corticosteroids)
- Idiopathic

AVN was classified by Ficat according to symptoms and the clinical and radiological findings. X-rays initially show no changes; however, after a few weeks reactive new bone forms in the adjacent living tissue, showing up as an increased area of density. Later on, the necrotic bone crumbles and the outline may be distorted. Bone scans show the region as an area of increased uptake due to the vascular reaction in the adjacent bone. The symptoms are usually pain and stiffness.

Idiopathic Avascular Necrosis (Osteochondritis)

In the earlier list the term "idiopathic" appears really for want of a better term. There is a group of conditions called osteochondritides, which are areas of patchy avascular necrosis of bone causing pain and limitation of movement, usually in adolescents. They are usually called by the names of those who described them, and examples include avascular necrosis of the second metatarsal head (Freiberg's disease), the navicular (Kohler's disease), the lunate (Kienbock's disease) and the capitulum of the humerus (Panner's disease).

The cause is unknown. There are two subgroups (traction apophysitis and osteochondritis dissecans), which still come under "osteochondritides", but because they have explainable causes they are listed here separately. Note that they are not inflammatory conditions and so the "itis" is not strictly correct.

Traction Apophysitis

Repetitive pulling forces of a tendon may damage the apophysis to which it is attached. The commonest example is the pull of the quadriceps on the tibial tuberosity, called Osgood–Schlatter disease (named after two separate surgeons who described the condition in the same year, 1903), which presents as knee pain, usually in growing adolescents. It is typically a self-limited condition that waxes and wanes, but which often takes months to years to resolve entirely, through stopping sports and conservative measures. In a small number of chronic cases where there is a bony ossicle in the patellar tendon, surgical excision is required and usually successful. Another example of traction apophysitis is Sever's disease of the calcaneus, due to the pull from the Achilles tendon.

Osteochondritis Dissecans

A piece of bone and its overlying articular cartilage may fall (dissect) off into the joint space due to repeated minor stresses. The commonest site is the knee, resulting in pain, swelling and limitation of movement. X-rays may show a loose body or a crater on the articular surface of the medial femoral condyle of the femur from which the fragment has fallen off.

Treatment depends on the size of the defect and the symptoms it causes. The options range from taking a "wait-and-see" policy to surgery which could include drilling, osteochondral autografting or autologous chondrocyte implantation. No good prospective randomised long-term trial results have been published to allow patients to make a really informed decision. A large defect will ultimately progress and lead to osteoarthritis, especially if located on the lateral femoral condyle.

BONE TUMOURS

This is not a common topic in finals, although you may be asked to write an essay or discuss this during a viva. Because there are so many types, students often learn them as a list and therefore do not know the relative importance of each type. In fact, all are incredibly rare, but you cannot be forgiven for not knowing two basic facts:

- Secondaries to bone are much more common than primaries.
- Primary bone tumours need to be managed by a specialist centre.

To learn about bone tumours, it is helpful to have a basic understanding of the terms used to describe bones, which cannot be understood without a brief introduction to the development of long bones. A bone begins life as a cartilaginous model of approximately similar shape to the final product into which it will be converted. The primary centre of ossification appears at the centre of the shaft or diaphysis (Greek for "in between") sometime during intrauterine life. The ossification spreads from here towards each end of the bone. Near the two ends of the bone there is a growth plate called the physis, from which longitudinal growth of the bone occurs initially as cartilage, which then undergoes ossification. At the outer end of the bone is the epiphysis (Greek for "on top") and this is also cartilaginous. Sometime after birth, a secondary centre of ossification appears at each epiphyseal end (Figure 15.14).

When you see an X-ray of a long bone of a child (depending on age), you see the ossified part of the epiphysis separated from the shaft by a gap. This is not actually a space but simply the unossified cartilaginous part of the bone known as the physis. From the physis, bone is laid down towards the diaphysis into an area of bone called the metaphysis (Greek for "next to"). As the ossification from the primary centre and that from the secondary centre meet, fusion of the growth plate is said to occur, indicating skeletal maturity.

Primary bone tumours can develop in any of the tissues that make up the bone. They can be benign (given the ending "-oma") or malignant ("-sarcoma"). If derived from bone they are called osteoid tumours, such as an osteoma or osteosarcoma. Similarly, if they are derived from the cartilage they are called chondromas or chondrosarcomas, and if they are derived from the fibrous tissue they are called fibromas or fibrosarcomas. You can get combinations of the two, e.g. osteochondromas. There are also tumours derived from the marrow,

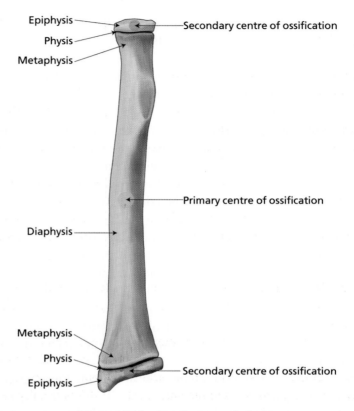

Figure 15.14.   Development of a bone.

including Ewing's sarcoma and myeloma. Some of the benign tumours can become malignant.

Symptoms from bone tumours usually include pain and swelling and certainly any such unexplained limb pain that lasts for more than a month (especially if pain occurs at night) should be investigated. The symptoms may be picked up incidentally on X-ray or present as a patho-logical fracture.

Most of the tumours have characteristic X-ray appearances; how-ever, there is a large amount of overlap and one X-ray appearance can have multiple differential diagnoses. The following X-ray appearances should be observed for warning signs of malignancy if noted on an X-ray.

- *Cortical destruction*. Is the cortical bone involved and eaten away? This can be a worrying sign.
- *Periosteal reaction*. This looks like a fuzzy line outside of the cortex, indicating activity or irritation of the periosteum. This is seen after a fracture or in infection, but can also be seen in their absence in the presence of malignancy.
- *Zone of transition*. These are the borders between the lesion and the normal bone. If the border can be drawn with a pencil (i.e. sclerotic margin) it is said to be a narrow zone of transition, which is less worrying than if the border is diffuse, which is associated with more aggressive tumours.

Other clinical indicators of malignancy include rapid growth of a lesion, tenderness and warmth (note that the latter two can also indicate infection).

If a malignancy is suspected, thorough investigation is needed to establish the exact diagnosis and assess the size and spread. Other investigations include a chest X-ray, bone scans, computed tomography (CT) and MRI. The erythrocyte sedimentation rate (ESR) is usually raised, as is the alkaline phosphatase. A biopsy should really be performed by the surgeon who will ultimately operate on the lesion, and therefore patients should be referred to a specialist centre early.

Primary Tumours

These should be thought of as benign or malignant. There are many differential diagnoses of benign tumours. It is beyond the scope of this book to cover every differential diagnosis in detail. Other texts do that very well. So below you will find some short notes that can be supplemented with further reading if you wish. For the purposes of exams it is fine that you have heard of the tumours listed; it is less important that you learn it off by heart as it is mainly postgraduate stuff.

Aneurysmal Bone Cysts (ABCs)

These are bone cysts that are expansile (hence their name). They usually affect those under the age of 30 and present with pain. On an MRI they display the pathognomonic sign of multiple fluid levels. Treatment of symptomatic bone cysts is usually to curette the cyst and fill with bone graft (Figure 15.15a)

Bone Cysts (Simple Bone Cysts or Unicameral or Solitary Bone Cysts)

Most of these occur in the proximal humerus and femur, again in young patients. They are usually asymptomatic but if they take up a large amount of the width of the bone they can fracture. If they do fracture, a bit of the cortex can fall into the cyst which gives the classical "fallen fragment sign".

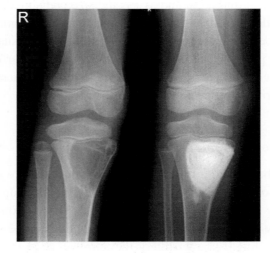

(a)

Figure 15.15.   Bone tumours: (a) an aneurismal bone cyst (ABC) before (image on left) and after curettage and filling (image on right).

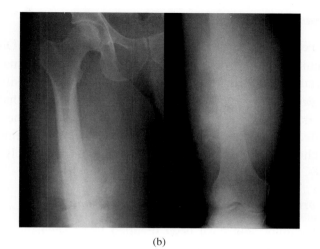

(b)

Figure 15.15. (b)   An osteosarcoma of the femur (note the expansile irregular mass that has broken through the cortex giving a "sun-ray" appearance).

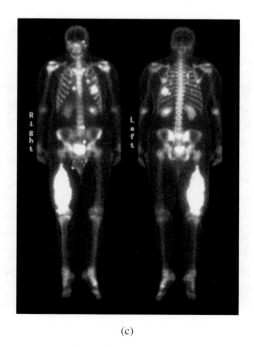

(c)

Figure 15.15. (c)   A bone scan of the same patient in 15.15b, showing increased uptake in the bone and surrounding tissues.

Chondromas (Enchondromas)

These are benign tumours which can be single or multiple (Ollier's disease). If multiple and associated with soft-tissue haemangiomas, there is another syndrome called Maffucci's syndrome, which we only mention for MCQ purposes as you are unlikely to ever see one. Chondromas or enchondromas are the most common benign cystic lesion of the phalanges but can affect other long bones. In patients over 40 it is important to exclude a chondrosarcoma, into which a chondroma can (rarely) develop.

Fibrous Cortical Defects (Non-ossifying Fibromas)

These are common and have been reported to be seen incidentally on X-ray in up to 20% of children. They usually spontaneously regress, however, and so are rarely seen after the age of 30. They are non-painful and benign defects of the cortex, as the name suggests, and usually affect the metaphysis of long bones. They should be left alone.

Fibrous Dysplasia

This is a condition whereby bits of the bone (usually long bones) are replaced by fibrous tissue. It can be monostotic (localised) or polyostotic (generalised). Monostotic is more common (approximately 70–80%). In monostotic fibrous dysplasia a solitary segment is affected and the cause is unknown. It is usually picked up incidentally on X-ray although it can present as a pathological fracture with pain.

In polyostotic fibrous dysplasia (20–30%) several bones are affected. It usually presents with progressive deformity (where the bones bend or enlarge), pain and pathological fracture. The classical X-ray appearance is described as a ground glass or smokey appearance. It has been questioned whether the Elephant Man had fibrous dysplasia, although most believe he had neurofibromatosis or Proteus syndrome.

There is a rare condition, worth a mention for a multiple choice exam, and that is McCune–Albright syndrome, which is where polyostotic fibrous dysplasia occurs in association with pigmentation of the skin (*café au lait* spots) and, in females, precocious puberty.

Giant Cell Tumours (GCTs)

These are sometimes called osteoclastomas and are of unknown origin, although there are multinuclear giant cells under the microscope, giving them their name. They occur in young adults, but always after fusion of the growth plate. If the growth plate is still open, discard this diagnosis. They are usually around the knee (in the lower end of the femur or upper tibia) and always abut the articular surface. They are usually considered benign neoplasms, although some can be locally aggressive and some metastasise.

Osteochondromas

These are the commonest tumours of bone. They are cartilage-capped exostoses that continue to grow as the bone grows (if multiple they may be part of a condition known as hereditary multiple exostoses). They usually present as a bony lump and appear on X-ray as an abnormal outgrowth of bone — either finger-like or cauliflower-shaped projections (often they look smaller on X-ray than they actually are, because the cartilage does not show up). If there are symptoms they should be excised, and if they change in size after skeletal maturity, then this suggests possible malignancy (chondrosarcoma).

Osteoid Osteomas

These are benign tumours that do not become malignant. They are small and usually occur in those under 30, most commonly in the tibia or femur. They appear on X-ray as a small radiolucent area (the nidus) surrounded by dense sclerosis and are hot spots on a bone scan. The main symptom is pain which characteristically responds to aspirin (but then again so do a lot of things). If left alone they may disappear spontaneously, but if the pain persists excision of the nidus may be undertaken, with instant resolution of the symptoms. Large osteoid osteomas have been referred to as osteoblastomas although they behave much like ABCs and if seen usually relate to the spine. We will not say any more as it's simply too rare for us to worry about.

A mnemonic to remember the list is "ABC FFG OO", if you are so inclined.

Malignant Tumours

Osteosarcomas

These occur in males more than in females, and usually in adolescents (although there is a second peak in those over 50, due to malignant change in Paget's disease). The commonest sites are around the knee or proximal humerus. Osteosarcomas usually occur in the metaphysis and are locally invasive, metastasising via the blood (often to the lung). The main symptom is pain, especially at night, and there may be local tenderness. X-rays show a metaphyseal, translucent and destructive lesion (Figures 15.15b and 15.15c). The tumour expands through the cortex, causing it to be raised, and a triangle of new bone is produced in the angle where the periosteum separates from the shaft, called Codman's triangle. Eventually it breaks through the cortex into the surrounding soft tissues, causing streaks of calcification within them (the "sun-ray" appearance). Treatment usually involves chemotherapy and resection, which may mean amputation or wide local excision using an allograft or prostheses. About 60% survive five years.

Ewing's Sarcomas

These are rare malignant tumours arising from the bone marrow, usually in young patients. Most of them occur in the diaphysis of long bones (in contrast to osteosarcomas which tend to be metaphyseal). Again, they present with a painful swelling, although because the lump is usually warm and tender they are occasionally diagnosed as having osteomyelitis. X-rays show a destructive lesion, sometimes with several layers of periosteal new bone around the lesion (called an "onion-skin" appearance). Treatment is usually chemotherapy, followed by surgical excision if possible.

Chondrosarcomas

These usually affect the middle-aged to elderly age group and are found in the pelvis or the proximal end of the long bones. There are two types: one arises from the surface of the bone (sometimes in the cartilage-covered cap of an osteochondroma) and the other arises within the medulla of the bone, often as a chondroma that either becomes malignant or has in fact been a slow-growing malignancy all the time. X-rays show an expanding radiolucent lesion with characteristic flecks of calcification. Treatment is by excision or, if necessary, amputation, since chondrosarcomas tend to metastasise late. Five-year survival is about 50%.

If the patient is young (less than 30) always think of an osteosarcoma or Ewing's sarcoma. In older patients (i.e. over 40) think of chondrosarcoma, myeloma and mets.

Secondary Tumours

Cancers that commonly metastasise to bone include breast, thyroid, renal, bronchus and prostate (not necessarily in this order, but it often helps to remember them by the mnemonic "Bone Tumours are Rarely Bony Primaries"). The majority of metastases are lytic lesions, with the exception of prostate, which is usually osteosclerotic. (However, breast and thyroid are sometimes osteosclerotic.) They metastasise to bone that contains red marrow, otherwise known as the axial skeleton (spine, pelvis, ribs and the proximal end of the long bones).

Secondary tumours may cause local pain or present as a pathological fracture. Pathological fractures are best treated by internal fixation, as they tend not to heal. By the time there are multiple bony secondaries the prognosis is poor and treatment is likely to be palliative. Radiotherapy is often used to treat local bone pain.

BONE INFECTION

Infection of bone (osteomyelitis) can be disastrous and extremely difficult to treat, and this is why such meticulous asepsis is undertaken in orthopaedic theatres and why antibiotic prophylaxis is always used when metalwork is involved. Acute osteomyelitis occurs either as a result of haematogenous spread or following trauma/operation. Infection of bones or joints acquired via the blood is common in children but rare in adults, who usually acquire the infection as a result of trauma or operation; the exception to this is in adults who are immunocompromised (including diabetics and those on steroids) or are intravenous (IV) drug abusers.

In acute haematogenous osteomyelitis, the usual organisms are *Staphylococcus aureus*, but occasionally streptococci or coliforms are responsible. They enter the blood in many ways, such as via a small skin abrasion or from an infected throat, and settle randomly on the bone. The symptoms usually include pain and fever, often with a preceding history of a sore throat or a superficial cut. The limb is painful to move, and there is tenderness and possibly localised inflammation. Diagnosis can be difficult in a young child, who may simply look unwell and have a temperature. X-rays are normal for the first week or so and later may show a hazy edge to the bone, indicating a periosteal reaction and new bone formation. A bone scan will show up increased activity while the X-rays are still normal.

Bloods should be sent for culture and white cell count, ESR and C-reactive protein (CRP), which should all be raised. Treatment is by IV antibiotics, analgesia and rest of the affected limb. The antibiotics are usually changed to oral after a few days and then given for up to six weeks.

Postoperative osteomyelitis where metalwork is *in situ* can be a disaster. Intravenous antibiotics are given and the metalwork may need to be removed and perhaps an external fixator applied if the fracture has not healed.

Chronic osteomyelitis can result if a sequestrum forms. A sequestrum is a piece of dead bone, often within a collection of pus. The pus can be walled off by new bone and might then discharge through a sinus. It can remain for many years, with intermittent flare-ups. An abscess within bone is known as a Brodie's abscess, named after Sir Benjamin Collins Brodie, 1st Baronet and surgeon to William IV and Queen Victoria. Surgery to remove the pus and sequestrum is indicated if healing is to ensue.

Acute Septic Arthritis

This usually affects large joints such as the hip in children and the knee in adults. The patient will feel unwell, often with a fever and rigors. The joint is painful, inflamed and swollen, and all movements are restricted.

X-rays may be normal initially and ultrasound may show a joint effusion. Diagnosis is based on clinical presentation but can only be confirmed by aspirating the affected joint under aseptic conditions and sending the aspirate to bacteriology for microscopy and culture. Blood tests should include an FBC, ESR, CRP and cultures (do not forget that tuberculosis can be a cause).

If your index of suspicion is high or the aspirate confirms sepsis, treatment involves joint washout under general anaesthetic and IV antibiotics. If there is a prosthesis *in situ*, then the infection may settle only if the metalwork is removed.

Sometimes it is difficult to make a diagnosis, for example when the patient has acute monoarthritis and the aspirate shows lots of white cells but no organisms. The differential diagnosis includes acute monoarthritis (rheumatoid), gout and pseudogout. However, clues from the history should help. For instance, does the patient feel generally well or unwell? Are they diabetic or on steroids? Have they had any previous episodes?

If the blood markers are all normal and the patient is apyrexial and looks well, septic arthritis is unlikely. They can be treated with splintage, rest and non-steroidal anti-inflammatory drugs. If there is any doubt in your mind as to the diagnosis, the safe option is to admit the patient for observation.

NERVE INJURIES

These are very common in finals and can appear both in medical and in surgical exams. When assessing the power of a particular muscle group, try to use the Medical Research Council classification, which scores power from 0 to 5; 5 is normal power, 4 is weakness, 3 is ability to use muscle against gravity, 2 is movement with gravity eliminated (for example, able to move in a horizontal direction but not vertically), 1 is just a flicker of muscle activity, and 0 means no movement detectable. It seems nonsensical to use plus or minus grades in a subjective scoring system, but no doubt you will see some people doing this.

Brachial plexus lesions can be of the upper or lower roots. The closer the lesion is to the spinal cord, the worse the prognosis will be.

Lesions of the upper brachial plexus (Erb's palsy, C5/C6) can occur at birth. Here the abductors and external rotators are paralysed, so the arm is held close to the body, internally rotated ("waiter's tip" position), with loss of sensation to the C5/6 dermatomes.

Lesions to the lower brachial plexus (Klumpke's paralysis, C8/T1) are rare and result in loss of intrinsic muscles of the hand, leading to a claw hand with loss of sensation in the C8/T1 dermatomes.

Injuries to the individual nerves of the arm can occur anywhere along the course of the nerve, and the deficit will depend on the level (Figure 15.16).

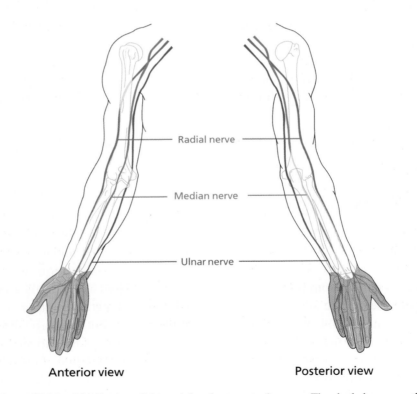

Radial nerve

Median nerve

Ulnar nerve

Anterior view   **Posterior view**

Figure 15.16.   Distribution of the peripheral nerves to the arms. The shaded areas on the hands correspond to the sensory distribution of each nerve.

Radial Nerve

The radial nerve is essentially the nerve which extends the fingers, the wrist and the elbow, and therefore testing the extension of each of these will give a clue as to the level. Sensation is not very accurate in helping to elicit the level, as it is predominantly a motor nerve.

Low lesions can occur with fractures around the elbow or forearm, and there is loss of extension of the carpophalangeal joints.

High lesions are more common and usually follow a fracture of the humerus or after a prolonged tourniquet time (the nerve is squashed or stretched but rarely severed). Damage usually occurs where the nerve travels around the shaft of the humerus (in the radial groove).

The patient has wrist drop, due to paralysis of the wrist extensors and loss of sensation along the radial nerve distribution (this is a common case in exams). Because the nerve to triceps comes off proximal to the lesion, the triceps still functions normally.

Very high lesions can be caused by pressure in the axilla such as through the incorrect use of crutches, or Saturday night palsy (the arm is hung over a chair when drunk). This leads to paralysis of the triceps as well.

Ulnar Nerve

Damage to the ulnar nerve usually occurs at the elbow or the wrist. The usual picture is a claw-like hand. The reason for this is that the ulnar nerve supplies all of the interossei, half of the flexor digitorum profundus (FDP) and the lumbricals to the ring and little fingers. A lesion at the wrist causes unopposed action of the extensors and the FDP, especially of the little and ring fingers, causing them to claw (the FDP is supplied just below the elbow and so a cut at the level of the wrist will not paralyse this).

Lesions at the elbow often lead to less clawing, since the ulnar half of the FDP is now paralysed and the fingers are therefore straighter (a true claw hand is only seen in Volkmann's contracture and proximal lesions of the brachial plexus).

Another test for the ulnar nerve is to ask the patient to grip a piece of paper between the thumb and the proximal phalanx of the index finger of a closed fist. In an ulnar nerve lesion the patient is unable to use the adductor pollicis, and to cheat they flex the DIPJ using the flexor pollicis (supplied by the median nerve) to grip the paper. If they flex the DIPJ, then this is called a positive Froment's sign.

The sensation in the ulnar distribution of the hand is usually affected. There may be wasting of the interossei on the dorsum of the hand, and there is weakness of finger abduction and adduction.

In an exam, if you see a wrist drop think of the radial nerve, and if you see a claw hand think of the ulnar nerve. Median nerve palsy is usually seen at the wrist, as in carpal tunnel syndrome.

Carpal Tunnel Syndrome

The median nerve supplies the first two lumbricals and the thenar eminence muscles. The muscles are often referred to as the LOAF muscles, which stands for Lumbricals (first two), Opponens pollicis, Abductor pollicis and Flexor pollicis brevis.

The median nerve can be compressed as it passes under the flexor retinaculum (in the carpal tunnel). It is much more common in females than in males and the associations are pregnancy, rheumatoid arthritis, hypothyroidism, acromegaly and trauma, although most often it is idiopathic in menopausal women.

The classic symptoms are pain and paraesthesia in the distribution of the median nerve (see Figure 15.16). A small patch of skin over the thenar eminence is spared, because this is supplied by the superficial branch of the median nerve, which does not go under the flexor retinaculum.

The symptoms of pain and numbness are classically worse at night and might be relieved by shaking the hands. During the day symptoms may be brought on by activities that compress the nerve further, such as prolonged flexion of the wrist (e.g. typing or knitting). In advanced cases the muscles supplied by the median nerve may be weak and wasted. Ideally, diagnosis should be made early from the history, before any physical signs are present, since once the muscle is wasted it invariably will not return even after a successful surgical treatment. A test that can sometimes reproduce the symptoms is Tinel's test (tapping over the median nerve at the wrist to reproduce the symptoms). The other test often associated with carpal tunnel is Phalen's test, where the wrists are held flexed for about 30 s (by pushing the dorsal surfaces of both hands together). This serves to increase the pressure in the carpal tunnel, increasing the pressure on the median nerve and exacerbating symptoms.

Always keep in mind a cervical rib or cervical spondylosis involving the C6 and C7 roots, which can cause similar symptoms, although the pain at night is really characteristic of carpal tunnel syndrome. If a case is suspected, diagnosis can be confirmed by electromyographic studies across the wrist showing delayed conduction of the nerve impulses.

Treatment of mild cases can be conservative, by using splints across the wrist or local steroid injections. Symptomatic cases where the nerve conduction is reduced require surgical decompression by division of the flexor retinaculum. The pain symptoms will improve; however, the numbness and wasting may not.

Dupuytren's Contracture

This is a common examination question. Named after the Frenchman who described it in 1931, Guillaume Dupuytren, it is a disorder where there is fibrosis and thickening of the palmar fascia (not the tendons!). It is commoner in men, usually of middle to elderly age. The aetiology is not known, although it can be inherited as an autosomal dominant gene. The associations include alcohol, drugs (such as phenytoin), cirrhosis and diabetes.

The condition often begins as a single nodule (which may or may not be painful). Later, bands of thickened tissue form on the palmar fascia which may adhere to the skin and there is progressive contracture of the fingers, usually the ring finger first, followed by the little finger, and eventually to the point where the fingers are fully flexed. The condition can be bilateral and the feet can sometimes be affected. Operation is considered for progressive lesions where the hand can no longer be placed flat on a table. It usually involves a fasciectomy, where the palmar fascia is divided. The condition can, however, recur. More recently new treatments have included needle fasciectomy (where the band is divided in an outpatient setting using a needle passed through the skin) or the use of an enzyme injection (collagenase clostridium histolyticum) in the outpatient setting. Widespread acceptance of these new techniques will require comparative clinical trials, none of which have yet been reported.

If you see a Dupuytren's contracture as a short case, the diagnosis is usually obvious although the differential diagnosis could include a skin contracture (an old laceration, scar or burn is, however, usually visible).

Ganglion

This is a common short case. A ganglion is a cystic swelling, most commonly seen on the dorsum of the wrist. Its exact origin is debated but is probably a cystic mucoid degeneration of the joint capsule or tendon sheath. It usually presents as a painless lump (but it can be painful) that may interfere with wearing a watch or may catch on clothes. A ganglion can disappear spontaneously, although a bash with a Bible was the traditional treatment. It is smooth and fluctuant and those at the wrist are usually fixed to deeper structures but not to skin. It can be aspirated (yielding a thick, gel-like material) and injected with hydrocortisone, although it commonly recurs, in which case it can be surgically excised.

Again the diagnosis is usually obvious, but the differential could be a lipoma, fibroma or sebaceous cyst.

THE LIMPING CHILD

Paediatric orthopaedics is a postgraduate subject and is not really considered fair game for surgical finals. The limping child is, however, an important subject and you should know a little about the following.

There is a diagnostic calendar of conditions that affect the hip and Table 15.2 illustrates the conditions and the rough age groups they tend to affect. The commonest cause of a painful hip in a young child is transient synovitis secondary to a viral illness, often called an irritable hip, but this is a diagnosis of exclusion.

Congenital Dislocation of the Hip (CDH)

At birth most hips are stable; however, a small number are dislocated or dislocatable. Most become stable within the first few weeks of life and

Table 15.2.   Diagnostic Calendar of Conditions

Age	Diagnosis	Rough incidence
0 (birth)	Congenital dislocation of the hip (CDH)	1 in 1000
0–5	Infections	
5–10	Perthes' disease (Legg–Calvé–Perthes)	1 in 10,000
10–15	Slipped femoral epiphyses	1 in 100,000
Adults	Avascular necrosis, rheumatoid and osteoarthritis	

can be considered to be physiological laxity of the joint capsule. The term "congenital dislocation of the hip" is used in many books to describe what is perhaps better classified as developmental dysplasia of the hip (DDH) because the problem is not always a dislocation and it is not always present at birth but can develop and progress during the first few months of life. Regardless of the name, it can be defined as a congenitally determined developmental deformation of the hip joint in which the head of the femur is or may be completely or partially displaced from the acetabulum.

The incidence of DDH is about 2 per 1000 live births although somewhere between 5–20 per 1000 hips are lax at birth. Females are affected more than males and one third are bilateral. The exact aetiology is unknown but there is a familial tendency and there is a high incidence of both joint laxity and a shallow acetabulum in first-order relatives of DDH patients. The position of the foetus in the uterus may play a part as there is a higher incidence in breech presentation, first-born children and those with oligohydramnios, all of which point to decreased intrauterine space.

It is also interesting to note that the incidence is much higher in North American Indians, who wrap their babies tight to the mother's body with the hips extended and the legs together, compared to the racially identical Eskimos, who carry their babies on the back with the hips widely abducted and flexed.

The best time to screen for DDH is at birth, during the routine postnatal examination. It is important for the screener to take a careful history, looking for risk factors for DDH, and obtain consent from the parents to carry out screening. On examination if there are any physical abnormalities (e.g. syndromic facies or scoliosis) this should be an additional warning sign. The buttock (gluteal) skin folds should be inspected and asymmetry should also set off alarm bells (asymmetry of inguinal skin folds is less helpful in the newborn although is significant in a 3–4-month-old baby).

Several tests have been described, of which the commonest described in the textbooks are the Ortolani and Barlow tests.

In Ortolani's test the hips and knees are flexed to 90° and the thighs are grasped in each hand, the thumb over the inner thigh and the fingers resting over the greater trochanters. The hips are abducted gently and resistance to abduction will be noted if the hip is dislocated; otherwise they abduct easily to 90°. When gentle pressure is applied to the greater trochanters by the fingers, a dislocated hip will relocate back into the joint and a click can be felt (positive Ortolani test). Barlow's test is a slight modification of this test. It is performed as above except during the abduction phase; gentle but firm pressure is applied in the line of the femur so that a lax hip dislocates posteriorly. The hip pressure can then be reduced by performing the movement in Ortolani's test. Therefore, one could think of the tests this way: Ortolani's test detects a dislocated hip and Barlow's test detects a dislocatable hip.

If either test is positive, or your clinical index of suspicion is high, then the baby should have an ultrasound scan. This will show the shape of the cartilaginous socket and the position of the head of the femur. X-rays are not helpful as the femoral head does not start to calcify until about ten weeks.

Treatment depends on the time of diagnosis, and generally the sooner the DDH is picked up the better the outcome. The actual treatments will vary from centre to centre but the principles of treatment are essentially the same, namely to reduce the hip and hold the head of the femur in this position until the acetabular rim is sufficiently developed.

Reduction can be obtained by closed or open methods. The younger the patient, the more likely that closed methods will be possible.

Closed Methods of Reduction

In the newborn this can be achieved initially with double nappies to abduct the hips, followed by a reassessment after 2–3 weeks with another ultrasound examination.

If the hip remains unstable it is possible to apply a special harness to hold the legs abducted. The most popular is called the Pavlik harness, which holds the legs in a position for a few months. It is imperative that the femoral head is shown to be in the right place using regular ultrasound.

If after another month the hip does not remain reduced using a spica, then it will be necessary to perform an examination under anaesthesia. There are higher anaesthetic risks in babies, so it is better to plan this electively when an experienced paediatric anaesthetist is available.

In theatre under general anaesthetic, an arthrogram (dye injected into the joint) is usually carried out to look for concentricity of the hip and any anatomical abnormalities. Because the abductors are likely to be tight, some surgeons will perform a tenotomy (where the tendon is cut) to allow gentle reduction, without excessive force which can damage the delicate blood supply to the hip. This is performed under image intensifier control. A plaster hip spica is then applied to keep the hip in the reduced position.

If the hip cannot be easily concentrically reduced, then an open reduction will need to be carried out. In very young children this is usually carried out at a later stage, when they are closer to a year old (because of the higher anaesthetic risks), and in the interim the hip is usually left untreated.

Open Reduction

The commonest open stabilising procedure is a derotation varus osteotomy of the femur. The leg is rotated to a position where the head has maximum covering in the acetabulum; the femur is then sawed just below the trochanters and the shaft allowed to rotate back to a neutral position, and the two ends are then fixed using a plate (e.g. Coventry screw plate).

Once in a good position the hip is held there using a plaster spica for a few weeks.

Once the toddler is walking the hip is checked regularly both clinically and radiologically and an assessment is made of the acetabular development. If unsatisfactory then further surgery may be required such as a pelvic osteotomy (the commonest is called a Salter osteotomy) to reposition the acetabulum to better cover the femoral head. This type of surgery is usually delayed until the child is about two years old.

If the diagnosis is not picked up at birth but picked up in the next few months, then the same principles apply. After about six months X-rays can be used to assess the acetabulum.

If the CDH is missed, then the diagnosis may not be made until the age of 12–18 months, when the child begins to walk with an abnormal gait. There may be limb shortening, external rotation of the foot, asymmetrical skin creases and a positive Trendelenburg's test. Reduction of the hip in this age group can be achieved by either open or closed methods as mentioned earlier (although a bit of labrum or loose capsule often impedes reduction and so closed reduction is usually unsuccessful).

The prognosis is good if the dislocation is picked up early, but if left untreated it can lead to progressive deformity and disability. Genetic testing can be discussed with the parents due to the familial tendencies.

With bilateral dislocations the deformity and waddling gait are symmetrical and not so noticeable; in fact such patients often carry on with their lives without much complaint. If you interfere with both sides you run the risk of one side failing and hence converting them to a unilateral asymmetrical deformity, and so most surgeons would not operate on such patients above the age of six.

Perthes' Disease

This is a type of osteochondritis, since it is an avascular necrosis of the femoral head. The patient is usually male, 4–10 years old, with a limp. Pain is dependent on the stage of the disease and although it initially may be painful, after a while it may become painless. If there is pain it is in the groin and may radiate down to the knee.

Early on all movements are painful, making it difficult to differentiate from infection or transient synovitis, which is by far the commonest cause of the irritable hip.

Initially X-rays are normal, although a bone scan may show an abnormality. The earliest change to be seen on X-ray is increased density of the bony part of the epiphysis, which later on flattens and fragments. A bone scan is useful especially in early stages of the disease.

There are at-risk signs (both clinical and radiological) that point to a poorer prognosis, although the details of these are perhaps more than you need to know for surgical finals.

Treatment is initially bed rest until the pain subsides, and further operative treatment will depend on the X-rays but essentially involves trying to contain the head in the acetabulum to enable it to retain as good a shape as possible.

Slipped Capital Femoral Epiphysis (SCFE)

Slipped capital femoral epiphysis in the past was referred to as slipped upper femoral epiphysis. It is an uncommon condition, usually found in children of pubertal age. It tends to affect two contrasting groups, one being the fat and sexually underdeveloped group and the other being the tall and thin group — boys more than girls.

Endocrine and mechanical factors might play a part, since fat children have a higher incidence. It has been proposed that SCFE is due to a hormonal imbalance at the time of a growth spurt.

The epiphysis slips posteriorly either as an acute event (acute slip — 20%) or over a period of time (chronic slip — 60%) or as a combination of the two (acute-on-chronic slip — 20%).

In an acute slip the patient usually presents with groin pain or pain referred to the thigh or knee. The leg may be slightly short, externally rotated, and initially all movements are painful. Treatment depends on the acuteness of presentation and the degree of displacement but usually involves surgery to reduce the epiphysis and hold it in place with a pin. In a chronic slip, reduction should not be attempted (as avascular necrosis may result) and the epiphysis is usually pinned where it is (*in situ*) to prevent further slippage.

One of the risks of SCFE you should know about is chondrolysis, where the articular cartilage breaks down. Although this can occur without surgery, the risk is higher if the guide wire or pin penetrates the articular cartilage.

In the longer term, all the hip disorders mentioned above can potentially increase the risk of disability, deformity and osteoarthritis.

Irritable Hip

This is a diagnosis of exclusion commonly made in children aged 1–10, and presents with a limp and pain in the hip. The cause is unknown but may be a viral synovitis as the patient often has a preceding upper respiratory tract infection. It is important to rule out septic arthritis, and so screening blood tests, including a FBC, CRP and ESR, must be sent off. An ultrasound examination may be helpful.

Infection in a joint can lead to destruction of the articular cartilage and permanent damage within a short space of time, and therefore a child in whom you suspect infection needs urgent aspiration of the joint to obtain microbiological samples for microscopy and culture. If there is no bacterial infection and an irritable hip is diagnosed, then it usually settles with rest and analgesia over 2–3 days.

16

EAR, NOSE AND THROAT

Philip Yates, Michael Oko and Ashraf Morgan

Ear, nose and throat (ENT) is an important subject and although examination questions are common they tend to be at a reasonably basic level in finals. Topics such as thyroid disease, dysphagia and lumps in the neck are important but are covered elsewhere in this book (Chapters 6 and 11).

OTOLOGY

Symptoms of Ear Disease

The specific symptoms that patients with ear disease complain of include the following.

Hearing Loss

Hearing loss is the most common symptom of ear disease, varying from mild through moderate, severe or profound. Hearing loss can be either conductive (where the abnormality is in the external or middle ear), sensorineural (where the abnormality is in the cochlear or auditory pathway) or mixed (a combination of both).

Discharge (Otorrhoea)

Discharge from the ear is usually secondary to infection of the auditory canal or middle ear. Mucopurulent discharge is likely to indicate origin from the middle ear through a perforation in the tympanic membrane, since there are no mucous-secreting glands in the auditory canal itself. A clear discharge after head injury can indicate cerebrospinal fluid (CSF) leak through a perforation in the tympanic membrane.

Pain (Otalgia)

As with discharge, infection of the auditory canal or middle ear is the commonest cause of pain. It is important to remember that pain can be referred to the ear from other areas such as the temporomandibular joint, teeth or pharynx (e.g. tonsillitis or even a malignancy in the pharynx).

Tinnitus

This is the subjective auditory sensation of noise without external sound stimulation (i.e. a sound heard when there is no sound present). Patients usually complain of a mechanical noise which is heard in both ears or centrally. Tinnitus is extremely common and can be associated with any form of hearing loss. Patients often complain their tinnitus is worse when they are in a quiet room (classically when trying to get to sleep), because there is no background noise to mask their tinnitus.

Less commonly, tinnitus is unilateral or pulsatile and this should arouse suspicion of underlying pathology. An example of pathology causing unilateral tinnitus is an acoustic neuroma. Pulsatile tinnitus could be caused by a vascular abnormality (e.g. glomus tumour).

Vertigo

This is the illusion of movement experienced by the patient. Often, though not always, vertigo originating in the vestibular system causes a sensation of rotation.

Examination of the Ear

Introduce yourself to the patient and pick up your auroscope. Choose an appropriately sized speculum to attach to the scope. (Make sure you are familiar with this instrument and can hold it properly, otherwise it might

be obvious to the examiner that you have never picked one up before!)
Ask the patient if they have a better hearing ear (unless directed to examine a specific ear by the examiner) and proceed to examine the better
hearing ear first.

Inspect the pinna (external ear) and surrounding skin using either a
headlight or the auroscope. Anteriorly look for preauricular sinuses and
any other congenital abnormalities such as an accessory auricle. Also look
for evidence of previous surgical incisions. An endaural incision is a surgical scar running from vertically just above the tragus (the bit of
skin-covered cartilage in front of the external auditory meatus). A postau-
ricular incision runs in the hidden groove between the back of the pinna
and the mastoid bone. These are often very subtle and can only be seen if
you look closely. It is useful to keep talking and explain to the examiner
what you are doing as you go along.

Once you have examined the external ear, gently pull the pinna pos-
terosuperiorly to straighten the ear canal and, holding the auroscope like
you would hold a pen, insert it into the external auditory canal. You should
usually hold it in the right hand to examine the right ear, and in the left
hand to examine the left ear. Remember that the speculum of the auroscope is used to push aside any hair in the lateral part of the ear canal. Do
not simply push the speculum as far into the ear canal as you can, as the
bony part of the external canal is extremely sensitive and you will hurt the
patient.

As an undergraduate you will not be expected to answer anything too
tasking with regards to abnormal findings within the ear canal or middle
ear. Demonstrating that you are familiar with how to use an auroscope to
examine the ear properly will often be sufficient.

If the ear canal is much wider than usual, it is likely the patient has
had surgery for a cholesteatoma, leaving a mastoid cavity. Look towards
the tympanic membrane (Figure 16.1) and look for the light reflex
anteroinferiorly (this is due to light bouncing off the conical-shaped tympanic membrane). Identify the handle of the malleus. Continue
examination of the pars tensa segment of the tympanic membrane and
note whether it is intact or not. If it is not intact, note what percentage of
the drum is perforated. In exams you would probably see a stable tympanic membrane perforation which is on a waiting list for elective surgery.

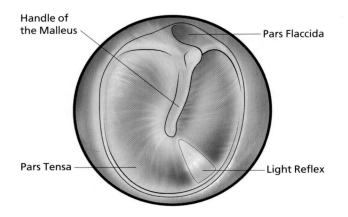

Figure 16.1.   Normal tympanic membrane.

Examine the pars flaccida (often referred to as the attic) and see if it looks retracted or if there any debris within it as this is the area in which a cholesteatoma often arises.

Do not forget to examine the function of the facial nerve and also the opposite ear. Free-field hearing tests are a useful conclusion to your inspection of the ear, so make sure your technique for this is good (see next section).

Hearing Tests

Tuning Fork Tests

A common question is to ask you to perform the Weber and Rinne tests. Always make sure you explain what you are going to do to the patient before you start. Strike the tuning fork on a bony prominence such as the elbow or knee. If the tuning fork is held with its base placed firmly on the skull, the sound is transmitted through the skull to the cochlea and sound is heard by bone conduction. If the fork is held near the pinna, sound is heard by air conduction. Classically a 512 Hz tuning fork is used because if you use a higher-frequency tuning fork the sound decays too quickly and if you use a lower-frequency tuning fork you get a lot of vibrational sensation.

Rinne Test

Explain that you will be tapping the tuning fork and placing it just outside the patient's ear, in front of the external auditory meatus (1), and then you will move it to their mastoid process and touch the skin/bone (2) (Figure 16.2).

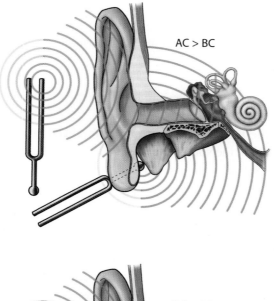

AC > BC

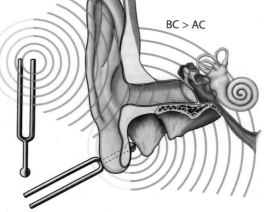

BC > AC

Figure 16.2.   Rinne test.

You then ask the patient to tell you which one was louder, 1 or 2, and repeat this on the opposite side. It is normal that air conduction (1) should be better than bone conduction (2) and this is a Rinne positive result. You can get a Rinne negative if bone conduction is better than air conduction due to a conductive loss. However, you can also get a false negative Rinne when the patient has a "dead" or non-functioning ear on the side being tested and they actually hear the tuning fork test in the opposite (normal) cochlea via bone conduction across the skull. It is hence necessary to carry out a Weber test alongside the Rinne test, especially when the Rinne test is negative, in order to determine whether it is a true or false negative result.

Weber Test

Gently strike the fork and place it on the forehead, asking the patient to confirm which side the sound lateralises. If the hearing is symmetrical the sound will not lateralise to one ear and will be perceived in the midline. With a unilateral conductive hearing loss, the sound will be perceived louder in the poorer hearing ear (towards the bad hearing ear). With a unilateral sensorineural hearing loss, the sound will be perceived in the better hearing ear (towards the good hearing ear) (Figure 16.3). Ambiguity develops when one ear has both conductive and sensorineural (mixed) hearing loss. You can remember this test by doing it on yourself, with one ear plugged with your finger to simulate a conductive loss.

Free-Field Hearing Tests

These are useful to know and if performed with confidence they look impressive in exams. Position yourself behind or to the side of the test ear so that lip reading is avoided. Test the better hearing ear first. Mask the non-test ear by gently occluding the auditory canal with a finger by rubbing the tragus. Start with a whispered voice at 2 ft (approximately an arm's length) using a combination of numbers and letters (e.g. "6C4"). If the patient correctly repeats the combination 50% of the time the hearing is considered normal. If the patient fails the test it can be repeated with a whispered voice at 6 in from the ear. If there is still inadequate response

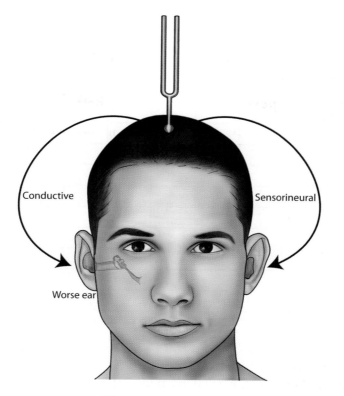

Figure 16.3. Weber test.

the above steps can be repeated with a normal conversational voice and finally a loud voice to give an idea of the severity of hearing loss.

Pure Tone Audiometry (PTA)

You may be expected to have heard of this and possibly interpret some of the most common results. An audiometer produces pure tones at several frequencies. The test is carried out in a soundproofed booth. The patient wears headphones connected to the audiometer. Tones are presented to the test ear at gradually reducing volume. Using this method the threshold of hearing can be determined at each frequency. A small vibrator can also be used, applied to the mastoid process, to assess bone conduction thresholds of hearing in a similar way. The threshold of hearing at different frequencies is

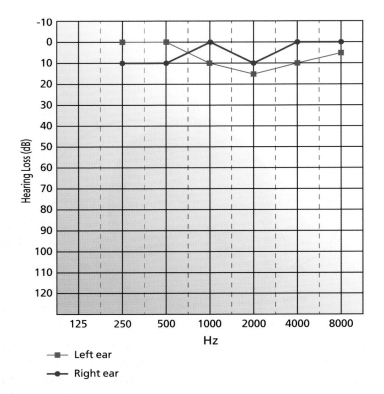

Figure 16.4. Normal audiogram.

plotted and this is the audiogram (Figure 16.4). Normal hearing is generally considered to be 20 dB or better.

Tympanometry

This is a simple but very useful test which is performed by inserting a probe into the ear canal. It measures the compliance (or stiffness) of the tympanic membrane. There are three common results from this test (Figure 16.5). If the middle ear pressure is equal to atmospheric pressure (normal) then a Type A curve is seen. If the middle ear pressure is negative in comparison to atmospheric pressure (usually due to Eustachian tube dysfunction) then a Type C curve is recorded. In the presence of fluid in the middle ear ("glue ear") then a flat Type B trace results.

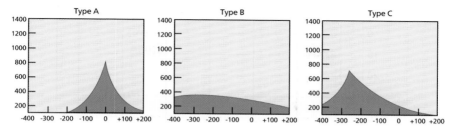

Figure 16.5.   Tympanometry.

Causes of Hearing Loss

As previously mentioned, hearing loss can be conductive, sensorineural or mixed. Each of these types of hearing loss can be congenital or acquired.

Congenital

Congenital hearing loss is present around the time of birth and the commonest cause is hereditary hearing loss which can be either non-syndromal (in which hearing loss is the only abnormality) or syndromal, such as Alport syndrome or Pendred syndrome (in which hearing loss is associated with anomalies in other systems). Other causes include intrauterine infections, such as cytomegalovirus (CMV) and rubella, and perinatal problems, such as hypoxia. It is worth noting that in England there is an NHS Newborn Hearing Screening Programme (NHSP), which offers all parents the opportunity to have their baby's hearing screened within the first few weeks of life.

Acquired

Adults

- *Ageing.* Presbyacusis (deafness of old age) is the most common cause of hearing loss in adults. Patients are usually over 65 years of age with bilateral sensorineural hearing loss of progressive onset over many years with or without tinnitus. There is a predominantly high-frequency "ski-slope" loss on PTA and the patient is treated by fitting hearing aids (Figure 16.6).

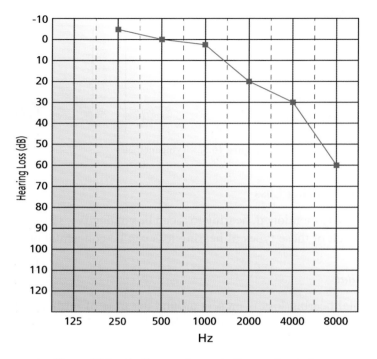

Figure 16.6.   Audiogram demonstrating presbyacusis.

- *Noise-induced hearing loss.* A history of long-term noise exposure at work is usual and may be associated with tinnitus. Classically, there is a high-frequency sensorineural hearing loss which is most pronounced at 4 kHz, producing a notch on the audiogram (Figure 16.7).
- *Otosclerosis.* This is a conductive hearing loss that is inherited in an autosomal dominant pattern with variable penetration. It presents with a progressive hearing loss, more commonly in women (with symptoms often being exacerbated by pregnancy). It is due to fixation of the stapes in the oval window and treatment is either with hearing aids or surgical replacement of the stapes with a prosthesis (stapedotomy).
- *Acoustic neuroma.* An acoustic neuroma is a benign neoplasm of the superior vestibular nerve and should correctly be referred to as a

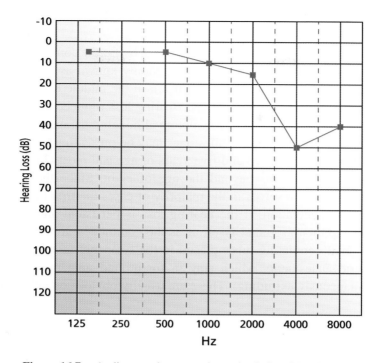

Figure 16.7. Audiogram demonstrating noise-induced hearing loss.

vestibular schwannoma, but its traditional name remains more popular. It usually presents with slow onset of unilateral symptoms of
hearing loss and tinnitus. Vertigo is rarely a symptom despite the fact
that it arises on the vestibular nerve. As the neuroma enlarges it can
also lead to brain stem compression and other cranial nerve palsies
(most commonly the trigeminal nerve). In view of this, patients with
unilateral hearing loss should always be referred for ENT assessment. In rare cases it presents bilaterally (e.g. neurofibromatosis
Type II). Investigation includes a full clinical exam, PTA (unilateral
sensorineural hearing loss) and magnetic resonance imaging (MRI)
scan. Because it is very slow growing, small tumours can be
observed by serial annual MRI scanning. If treatment is required the
options are either stereotactic radiotherapy (Gamma Knife) or
surgical removal.

Children

- *Otitis media with effusion (OME).* This is by far the commonest cause of hearing loss in children. It is commonly known as glue ear. It is defined as a serous or mucoid effusion in the middle ear which persists for more than three months. Hearing loss (noticed by parents or teachers) is usually the only symptom although poor speech development and other abnormal milestones may be presenting features. The incidence peaks at two and five years of age and most children have no further problems beyond the age of eight. Since the condition spontaneously resolves in the majority of cases the first line of treatment is observation. If the hearing loss is persistent and causing a handicap then grommet insertion is the commonest treatment (these are small ventilating tubes placed in the tympanic membrane under general anaesthetic, which stay in for around nine months before spontaneously extruding). These are usually obvious on auroscopy.

Common Conditions of the External Ear

Pinna

Remember to look for evidence of congenital abnormalities when examining the external ear (e.g. in the pinna you would look for an accessory auricle, preauricular sinuses, microtia). Also remember that some congenital abnormalities of the ear may be associated with syndromes such as Treacher Collins.

Trauma to the pinna can result in a haematoma of the pinna and if this is not drained it will often result in a "cauliflower ear". Because of the exposed position of the pinna it is prone to sunlight exposure and hence the skin is at risk of malignant changes. Basal cell carcinoma, squamous cell carcinoma and malignant melanoma can all affect the pinna, particularly in countries where exposure to prolonged sunlight is more common.

Conditions of the External Auditory Canal

The most common condition affecting the external auditory canal is chronic otitis externa, which is treated with aural toilet (clearing of the infected debris from the ear canal) and a topical antibiotic, commonly gentamicin ear drops. Response to oral antibiotics is usually poor.

Malignant otitis externa is a misnomer as it is not a neoplastic condition. The name arises from its high mortality rate in the past. In immunocompromised individuals, particularly elderly diabetics, infection of the ear canal can cause osteomyelitis of the skull base. Symptoms or signs that should raise your suspicion include the following: otitis externa failing to respond to treatment; associated severe pain; and associated lower cranial nerve palsies. Malignant otitis externa usually responds to prolonged treatment with systemic antibiotics such as tazocin.

Bony exostoses can also appear in the exam and they usually present as smooth symmetrical bony swellings of the external auditory canal in people who do a lot of swimming in cold water (such as surfers). Treatment is conservative unless it is significantly problematic, then drilling away the bony exostosis can be performed. Malignancy of the ear canal is extremely rare.

Middle Ear Infections

Acute Otitis Media

This is one of the most common infections in children, most commonly presenting around two years of age. Although you are unlikely to see a patient with this condition in the exam you could be shown a picture of an acutely inflamed eardrum. A child crying in pain, a history of an upper respiratory tract infection associated with fever, and ear discomfort should make you suspicious of this common condition. When you look at the tympanic membrane it is usually acutely inflamed and bulging. If the tympanic membrane ruptures there will be a mucopurulent discharge. Usually the infection settles quickly after the pus drains and the perforation heals. Treatment consists of analgesia (usually paracetamol) and antibiotics (such as amoxicillin) if the condition does not resolve after a day or two. The main concern with acute otitis media that does not respond to treatment is that it can be complicated by meningitis or acute mastoiditis. Acute mastoiditis is an osteitis of the temporal bone with abscess formation which often requires a surgical mastoidectomy to drain the pus.

Perforation of the Tympanic Membrane

Perforation of the eardrum is most commonly due to repeated episodes of acute otitis media with perforation. Usually the patient presents with repeated or recurrent infection with discharge and an associated hearing loss. If symptoms are problematic the perforation can be repaired surgically (myringoplasty).

Cholesteatoma

Although this condition sounds as though it is a neoplasm it is in fact simply a retraction in the tympanic membrane (usually the pars flaccida) which gradually expands and fills with desquamated squamous epithelium which is prone to infection. These patients present with a persistent smelly discharge from the ear which is almost always associated with hearing loss due to destruction of the ossicles. If left untreated this condition carries a high risk of causing meningitis or a brain abscess, and hence a cholesteatoma is almost always removed surgically (mastoidectomy), unless the patient is unfit or refuses surgery.

Vertigo

Although patients with a balance disorder can be complicated to unravel, they could certainly be used as an exam case. The history is key to diagnosis. It is important to remember that balance relies upon input from vision (70%), proprioception (15%) and the vestibular system (15%). Often patients will have multiple medical contributions and be on lots of medications that could contribute to a balance disorder. Vestibular disorders that can result in vertigo have specific features in the history:

Benign Paroxysmal Positional Vertigo (BPPV)

This condition presents with short-lived (seconds) of rotational vertigo precipitated by certain head movements, classically turning over in bed. It is due to loose debris in one of the semi-circular canals which stimulate the sensory epithelium when disturbed. The diagnosis can be confirmed by performing a Dix–Hallpike manoeuvre which will reveal torsional nystagmus when the patient is laid back with the head extended. The condition can be cured by an Epley manoeuvre which moves the debris to an area where it does not cause symptoms.

Acute Vestibular Failure (Labyrinthitis)

This condition is thought to be viral in origin. It presents with a sudden onset of severe vertigo often associated with nausea and vomiting. Symptoms are usually present for several days before they subside. Treatment is with a vestibular sedative such as prochlorperazine. Usually vestibular function does not recover and so elderly patients may be left with a feeling of disequilibrium.

Ménière's Disease

This condition is defined as episodic vertigo associated with hearing loss and tinnitus. Often the patient has a preceding fullness in the affected ear. Symptoms last for several hours. As the vertigo subsides, the hearing loss and tinnitus resolve. It is thought to be due to fluctuations in the pressure in the endolymph (hence the alternate name of endolymphatic hydrops). Because the patient has a unilateral sensorineural hearing loss an MRI is performed to exclude an acoustic neuroma as the cause. The condition generally runs a chronic course for several years and finally burns out with complete loss of hearing in the affected ear. Many conservative, medical and surgical treatments are available for Ménière's disease but results are variable. In severe cases surgical labyrinthectomy or vestibular nerve section may be required.

Disorders of the Facial Nerve

The facial nerve enters the temporal bone through the internal auditory meatus and runs on the medial wall of the middle ear before entering the neck through the stylomastoid foramen. It enters the substance of the parotid gland before dividing into its terminal branches to supply the muscles of facial expression. Note that upper motor neuron lesions of the facial nerve spare the forehead whereas lower motor neuron (LMN) lesions do not (this is because of suprapontine crossover and sharing between the two sides). The facial nerve should be tested by asking the patient to lift their eyebrows, close their eyes tightly, purse lips and blow, and show you their teeth, which will reveal function in the important branches.

Bell's Palsy (Idiopathic Facial Nerve Palsy)

Bell's palsy is an LMN lesion of unknown cause, but possibly viral. It is a diagnosis of exclusion and a full clinical examination needs to be completed to exclude other causes. Treatment with a short course of high-dose steroids within 24 h of onset is generally recommended. In practice, full recovery may be expected in the majority of cases.

Herpes Zoster Oticus (Ramsay Hunt Syndrome)

This is a syndrome of LMN facial palsy associated with herpes zoster (shingles) affecting the ear. Recovery rates are much lower in this condition compared to Bell's palsy (approximately 50%).

Other Causes

Don't forget that malignant parotid lumps may cause a facial paralysis but if you get one of these in the exam it will usually be obvious. Trauma to the temporal bone with a skull base fracture can lead to a complete LMN facial palsy. In about 5% of cases the facial nerve is exposed as it passes through the middle ear and hence acute otitis media, which puts pressure on the unprotected nerve, or cholesteatoma can (rarely) lead to LMN facial nerve palsy. Mastoid surgery can cause iatrogenic facial nerve palsy, so it is important to look for evidence of surgical scars or a mastoid cavity in a patient with a long-standing facial palsy.

RHINOLOGY

Symptoms of Nasal Disease

The function of the nose is to warm, humidify and filter inspired air before it reaches the lungs. The symptoms to specifically ask about in the history of a patient with nasal problems are as follows:

Obstruction

Obstruction can be persistent, such as with nasal polyps, or may be seasonal, suggesting an allergic aetiology.

Discharge (Rhinorrhoea)

Nasal discharge can be clear, purulent or blood-stained. Watery discharge is seen in the elderly and patients with allergy, but can also be due to CSF leak (although rarely). Infection in the nose and sinuses is almost always associated with discharge.

Sense of Smell

Loss of sense of smell can be complete (anosmia) or partial (hyposmia). Since taste is dependent on the ability to smell, the patient may complain primarily of loss of taste. Anosmia is relatively rare and usually follows a viral infection or head injury (which shears the olfactory nerves at the cribriform plate).

Facial Pain

Facial pain may be associated with sinusitis along with other nasal symptoms. Facial pain with no associated nasal symptoms is often misdiagnosed as sinusitis when in fact it is a form of headache or neuralgic pain.

Bleeding (Epistaxis)

See below.

Examination of the Nose

This would be an uncommon question for finals, but simple to learn, so it is worth a brief description. Introduce yourself to the patient. Look directly at the nose from the front, side and from above. The upper half of the external nose is bony and the lower half is cartilaginous. By covering each part of the nose alternately it is possible to determine whether any deviation seen is bony, cartilaginous or both.

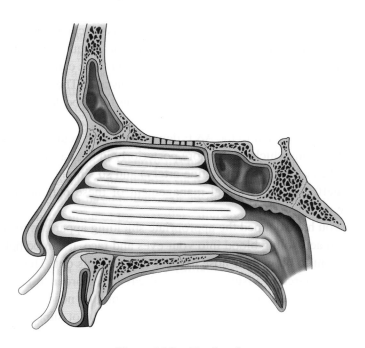

Figure 16.8.   Nasal pack.

exclude any other pathology such as nasal polyps. Skin prick allergy tests
or radioallergosorbent test (RAST) serology can be used to test for a wide
variety of common nasal allergens. The mainstay of treatment is allergy
avoidance, antihistamines (orally or topically) and/or topical nasal steroids.
The use of topical steroids requires caution in children, particularly if they
are using steroid inhalers for asthma, as they can cause growth delay.

Rhinosinusitis

Acute bacterial sinusitis usually develops following an upper respiratory
tract infection. It is characterised by a dull localised pain over the affected
sinus, often exacerbated by bending forwards. The pain is associated with
nasal obstruction and mucopurulent discharge. Treatment consists of nasal
decongestants and analgesia. If symptoms do not settle, a course of antibiotics is indicated. Acute sinusitis can be complicated by spread of

infection into the orbit, leading to periorbital cellulitis and abscess formation. If the abscess is not drained urgently, there is a risk of permanent damage to vision.

HEAD AND NECK

Symptoms of Disease in the Pharynx and Larynx

Pain

A sore throat is usually due to an infection of the pharynx, most commonly viral. Persistent pain, particularly if it is unilateral and present on swallowing (odynophagia), may be indicative of a pharyngeal cancer. Pain in the throat may be referred to the ear.

Dysphagia

This is difficulty swallowing and is dealt with in Chapter 6.

Hoarseness (Dysphonia)

See section on benign laryngeal disease.

Stridor

This is noisy respiration due to obstruction at the level of the larynx or below and may be inspiratory, expiratory or biphasic.

Stertor

This is noisy respiration due to obstruction at the level of the tonsils and tongue base, for example snoring.

Neck Lump

A patient may complain of having noticed a lump in the neck. Neck lumps are discussed in Chapter 11.

factors, oral cancers are uncommon. Oral cancer may be preceded by areas of leukoplakia and proceed to painful ulceration, possibly with associated cervical lymphadenopathy.

Tonsillar Malignancy

Cancers of the tonsils are usually due to either lymphoma or squamous cell carcinoma. Lymphoma tends to present as a unilateral swelling of the tonsil with associated lymphadenopathy. Squamous cell carcinoma is usually associated with a history of smoking and alcohol consumption, although more recently infection with human papillomavirus has been associated with tonsil carcinoma in non-smokers, and carries a better prognosis.

Nasopharyngeal Carcinoma

This is a rare cancer (although it is more common in the Chinese) which can present with nasal obstruction, unilateral glue ear or simply as a neck lump due to metastasis.

Diseases of the Larynx

The primary function of the larynx is to protect the airway from aspiration of food or liquid during swallowing. It also is essential for the production of voice.

Benign Laryngeal Disease

Hoarseness is the most common symptom of laryngeal disease. Laryngitis is an inflammation of the larynx, usually due to infection. In the majority of cases it settles quickly and the voice recovers. Occasionally, inflammation persists and results in chronic laryngitis.

Vocal cord nodules, often called singer's nodules, are symmetrical swellings on the vocal cords due to chronic voice (ab) use. They usually settle with voice therapy.

Vocal cord polyps are rare and tend to follow an acute infective episode. They require surgical removal. Recurrent respiratory papillomas can cause hoarseness, usually presenting in childhood.

Malignant Laryngeal Disease

Hoarseness can be due to malignancy in the larynx or malignancy in the chest invading the recurrent laryngeal nerve and causing a vocal cord palsy. For this reason a chest X-ray should be considered for a smoker with persistent hoarseness. As with other head and neck malignancies, laryngeal cancers tend to be squamous cell carcinomas and are associated with a history of smoking and drinking.

Since the left recurrent laryngeal nerve has a longer course in the chest, looping around the arch of the aorta (compared to the right side where the nerve loops around the subclavian artery), left-sided bronchogenic carcinoma is more frequently associated with hoarseness, due to vocal cord palsy.

Treatment of laryngeal cancer may require surgical removal, radiotherapy or chemotherapy, or a combination of these modalities.

PAEDIATRIC AIRWAY ISSUES

Congenital Abnormalities

Laryngomalacia

This is the commonest cause of stridor in infants. Inspiratory stridor typically develops a few days or weeks after birth and is initially mild, but over the ensuing months becomes gradually more pronounced, usually peaking at the age of 6–9 months. Typically, symptoms are worse during sleep, stridor being worse when the patient is in the supine position and improved when the patient is prone. Both feeding and exertion tend to result in more pronounced stridor. The epiglottis is classically described as being omega-shaped and folded in upon itself so that the lateral margins lie close to each other (Figure 16.9). A flexible nasendoscopy under local anaesthetic is usually carried out, proceeding on to a microlaryngoscopy and bronchoscopy (MLB) to confirm the diagnosis. Treatment is usually conservative but surgical epiglottoplasty is highly effective in appropriate cases.

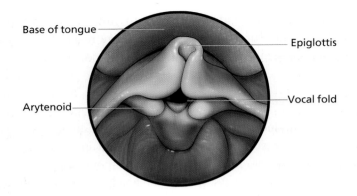

Figure 16.9.   Appearance of the infantile larynx in laryngomalacia.

Acquired Abnormalities

Acute Laryngotracheobronchitis (Croup)

Laryngotracheobronchitis is the most common infectious cause of airway obstruction in children, usually occurring between the ages of six months and three years. It is a viral infection most commonly caused by the parainfluenza virus. Characteristically, the symptoms of laryngotracheobronchitis are gradual in onset and are often preceded by an upper respiratory tract infection. A barking cough is invariably present along with hoarseness and stridor. If stridor is present, it is usually inspiratory in nature, and the onset of biphasic stridor and other signs of respiratory distress are indicative of severe airway obstruction. Symptoms typically last 3–5 days, although the child may be infectious for two weeks. Over 85% of cases of laryngotracheobronchitis are mild and can be managed in the community. In patients with more severe symptoms, nebulised epinephrine produces a rapid improvement in symptoms and steroids have a delayed but prolonged effect.

Acute Epiglottitis (Supraglottitis)

Typically, acute supraglottitis presents in children aged 2–6 years, although any age group, including adults, can be affected. *Haemophilus influenzae* Type B (HIB) is the responsible pathogen in most cases, and as a result of the introduction of the HIB vaccine, the incidence of epiglottitis has been reduced by more than 90%. Although it is a rare infection, awareness of the disease is important because of its high mortality rate (if not promptly diagnosed and treated). Symptoms progress rapidly over a matter of hours. The typical features are fever, difficulty in breathing and severe odynophagia, resulting in drooling. Inspiratory stridor is a late feature occurring when the airway is almost completely obstructed. Once the diagnosis of supraglottitis is suspected, further investigations should not be undertaken since any procedures that induce anxiety in the patient, including intraoral examination, may precipitate complete airway obstruction.

The management of a child with suspected supraglottitis requires close cooperation between the otolaryngologist, anaesthetist and paediatrician. The child should be directly transferred to theatre where equipment for emergency tracheotomy must be available. After inhalational anaesthesia, the supraglottis can be inspected and the presence of erythema and oedema confirms the diagnosis. The airway is then secured by endotracheal intubation. Once the airway is safe, blood cultures and swabs of the supraglottis can be obtained and an intravenous cannula inserted. Parenteral antibiotic therapy (e.g. ceftriaxone or cefotaxime) should then be started.

Foreign Body

Most inhaled foreign bodies pass through the larynx and trachea and become lodged distally. There is often a history of the child having something in the mouth before the onset of symptoms. If a foreign body becomes lodged in the larynx and causes complete obstruction, it will cause sudden death unless removed immediately. If the airway is only partially obstructed, then stridor, hoarseness and cough are the predominant symptoms. If the object is radio-opaque, its site of impaction can be confirmed by X-ray. Removal under general anaesthesia is generally required.

Subglottic Stenosis

Although subglottic stenosis can be congenital, it is more commonly acquired due to prolonged intubation. The subglottis is the narrowest portion of the airway in children, and the cricoid cartilage is the only complete cartilaginous ring in the airway. The degree of stenosis dictates the severity of stridor. Severe congenital subglottic stenosis presents at birth with stridor and respiratory distress. Less severe stenosis is likely to present in the first few months of life when increased activity requires increased respiratory efforts. The subglottic oedema produced by upper respiratory tract infections often precipitates stridor, which leads to misdiagnosis of recurrent laryngotracheobronchitis. Treatment depends on severity and ranges from observation, if mild, to resection and reconstruction, if severe. A tracheostomy may be required to ensure that the airway is safe until laryngeal reconstruction can be planned.

17

THE EXAM

Andy Goldberg, Gerry Stansby and Ben Bannerjee

Examinations are formidable even to the best prepared, for the greatest fool may ask more than the wisest man can answer.

C. C. Colton

Most medical schools set a mixture of written, viva voce and clinical examinations. Written papers are usually single best answer multiple choice questions (MCQs) or extended matching questions (EMQs). In some centres you might still be asked short answers or essays, although they are much less common nowadays. It is important that you know the format of your exam and what will be covered — so it's worth getting a copy of the syllabus early on.

Clinical exams usually consist of short cases, long cases or both. In some medical schools, medical and surgical cases are examined together and this is becoming more common. In others, surgical cases are examined in a separate section of the exam. It is important that you understand how the exams run in your own medical school, as it will influence the way you should prepare for them. In addition to getting the syllabus, you should also speak to people who have done the exams in previous years and look through as many past papers as possible.

Each year at medical school the majority of students pass their finals. Essentially, the aim of the examiners is to vet out anyone who is unsafe to be a junior doctor (Foundation Year 1). It is a bit like a game with hard and fast rules. If you abide by the rules of the game you will pass, and if you break them you will be penalised and could fail. The following list includes some of the rules to abide by, to avoid failing finals:

- Dress smartly and look respectable.
- Be polite to the patients (or actors) and try to build a rapport, because if they don't like you they could land you in difficulty.
- Never hurt the patients (or actors).
- Never make anything up and never say anything dangerous. If you do not know something a good option is to say that you would ask a senior for advice. For a particular drug you could say that you would look it up in a drug formulary, for example the *British National Formulary* (BNF).
- Wash your hands before any physical examination and ensure that your nails and hands are well groomed.
- The examiners are always right — do not answer back and do not argue.

If the examiners think that you would be unsafe as a junior doctor then they will fail you. Know the management of emergency conditions well because if your viva is not going well the examiners will usually change the subject to one that you should know something about in order to be a safe doctor. For example, you should know the emergency management of a shocked patient. If you say that you would order a CT scan before saying that you would place two large-bore cannulae into the antecubital fossae and start fluids, then you deserve to fail.

CLINICAL EXAMINATION

You should be smartly dressed and arrive early. The clinical examination is often the most worrying part of the exam for students. It can be quite difficult to think clearly in such a high-tension situation and it is important that you have prepared your basic history-taking and examining techniques in advance so that you can perform these on autopilot and concentrate specifically on your answers to the examiners. One of the best ways to prepare yourself is by practising with your colleagues or with medical staff at the firms you are attached to. It is possible for you to work efficiently for much longer periods when revising and practising together.

Viva Voce Examination

This usually takes the form of the candidate sitting at a desk opposite two examiners. Topics can cover any area of surgery, and sometimes X-rays, specimens or surgical instruments may be shown. In some medical schools the viva is the last part of the exam and commonly the examiners will know something of the candidate's performance by that point. In other medical schools the viva is only held for deciding who should get a distinction or for those with borderline marks who are in some danger of failing.

The examiners quickly develop an overall impression of you; therefore, it is important not to ponder far too long on the first question asked. If you do not understand a question, after a short period of reflection tell the examiners that you do not understand and ask them to rephrase the question. If you do this they will usually give some extra information or a hint to help you in the correct direction. This is much better than simply asking them to repeat the question where you will probably get no extra information and will still be unable to answer.

Always try to classify your answer in a logical way (e.g. the surgical sieve). Start with the simpler and more common things and work to the more complex and rarer elements. Remember, if the questions appear to be getting harder this usually means you are doing well, as the examiners need to assess how good you are, so that they can give you a grade. Most people leave the room only remembering the last question asked — which is, as explained, usually the most difficult. This is why you should never ask the candidate leaving the viva before you what they were asked.

Objective Structured Clinical Exams (OSCEs)

Many medical schools now use OSCEs as part of their examinations. The principle of these is to provide uniformity in the exam for all students and not have the unpredictabilty that is inherent in the standard clinical exams. There is usually no negative marking in an OSCE.

Since all candidates will be examined on the same material, it is possible to unify marking across examiners in a way that would not otherwise be possible. Often actors are used instead of real patients. The usual approach for an OSCE exam is to have a number of stations at which the candidate has to carry out tasks. For example, one station might be to carry out an abdominal exam, another to consent a patient for a colostomy, etc. Examiners may be present to mark the candidate, which can sometimes be off-putting; however, they would not normally speak or question the candidate directly. Some stations may also consist of X-rays with a list of questions or pictures of clinical signs, etc., where the candidate completes an answer sheet which is marked afterwards. Where actors are used they are usually asked to give out only one piece of information at a time. For example, the question "Do you have abdominal pain?" would produce the answer "Yes" and you would then have to ask "Where is the pain?" as a separate question.

There is nothing inherent in an OSCE which should trouble the well-prepared candidate. One problem may be completing the task within the time allowed at each station, and you should therefore find out the format of the exam well in advance and practise doing things to time.

Short Cases

These were traditionally used in most medical schools but have been pretty much replaced by OSCEs nowadays. A large number of cases, usually with physical signs, are assembled together in one place. The candidate is taken from case to case by the examiners.

The examiners usually work in pairs, with one questioning and the other marking. Do not be put off by this. There is no truth in the commonly held belief that you have to get through a particular number of short cases to be able to pass. Remember to briefly introduce yourself to the patients, ask them if they mind you examining them and make sure you preserve their dignity but without compromising on exposure. Most marks will be awarded for using the correct technique of examination and not necessarily for reaching a diagnosis. Not all short cases will take the same length of time to deal with. If the case is very straightforward (for example, a case of Dupuytren's), simply state the features and diagnosis so that the examiners can either move on or ask you extra questions about treatment, etc. Above all, be guided by the examiners as to what you should examine and how quickly.

Common short cases include the following:

- Neck lumps (especially thyroid)
- Groin lumps (especially hernias and testicular lumps)
- Hands (Dupuytren's, ganglions and nerve lesions)
- Skin cancers and lumps (e.g. basal cell carcinomas, lipomas and neu-fibromas)
- Abdominal examinations (enlarged liver or stomas)
- Lower limbs (varicose veins, anterior cruciate ligament tears, knee osteoarthritis or chronic ulcers)
- Feet (hammer toes, hallux rigidus or hallux valgus)

Long Cases

Most medical schools expect the candidate to be examined on a surgical long case. The principle of the long case is that the candidate is left alone with the patient to take a history and carry out an examination. Leave 5 min at the end to quickly gather your thoughts on how you are going to present the case to the examiners. The time allowed with the patient varies enormously (20–60 min). In medical schools where 1 h is allowed, this is usually enough time for a full standard history and examination, and time itself should pose no problem. When the time available is shorter, the candidate may have to limit the history and examination to the most important points. This will be understood by the examiners, and if asked about something you did not have time to do, you must state this clearly. It is a fatal error to waffle or, even worse, make something up. Remember also that the examiners may take you back to the case and go over the points in question with you. If you are found to have made something up, then usually you will automatically fail this part of the exam. If possible, present the case without looking at your notes continuously (sample presentations are given in this chapter). Eye contact with the examiners will help to make a good impression.

Common long cases include abdominal operations (e.g. postoperative bowel resection for cancer or inflammatory bowel disease), vascular cases (carotid disease, aortic aneurysm or peripheral vascular disease), orthopaedic cases (joint replacements for osteoarthritis) and breast lumps (usually elderly patients).

When you present your long case to your examiner, have a provisional diagnosis or differential in mind. It is sometimes possible to predict what questions the examiner is going to ask you, and it will help if you have thought of the answers before the questions are asked. Leave 5 min at the end of your clerking to get your ideas together and to write a quick summary.

WRITTEN PAPERS

For most written papers we would recommend the following:

- Read the instructions at the top of the paper carefully (i.e. how many questions should be answered, time allowed, etc.). Do not presume that they will be the same as for past papers you may have looked at during your revision. If you are not sure, ask the invigilator, who is there for that purpose.
- Calculate exactly how much time should be spent on each question after allowing 5 min for reading the paper.
- Slowly read each question in turn, until you are sure you understand what the questions are asking.
- Consider writing a rough plan/bullet points for each answer. Use the surgical sieve to prevent yourself from forgetting anything.
- Spend only the amount of time allowed on any one question.
- On no account fail to answer a question. If the worst happens and you run out of time, hand in your plan/bullet points.

Multiple Choice Questions (MCQs)

Multiple choice exams can be negatively marked (i.e. one mark is given for a correct answer, nothing for an answer not attempted and one mark is taken away for an incorrect answer) or not negatively marked (i.e. one mark is given for a correct answer and no marks for an incorrect answer or one not attempted).

In negatively marked exams, guesswork is unlikely to improve your marks and may in fact reduce them. If possible, clarify what type of marking scheme is used in your medical school well in advance of the exam.

We suggest you approach MCQs in the following way:

- Calculate the time available and aim to go through the paper in 60% of that time.
- Go through the questions, answering only those you are fairly certain you know the answers to.
- Go back over the questions you have not answered and see if there are any that you can now answer with a fair degree of certainty.
- Questions using the words "always" and "never" are invariably false; likewise, questions using the word "may" are usually true (for example, "Vomiting is always present in bowel obstruction" would be false).
- Make sure you spend a moment on each question considering the exact wording and sense of the question — this can make a big difference in the multiple choice. For example, "Perforated peptic ulcer is always treated by operation" is not the same as "Perforated peptic ulcer is usually treated by operation".
- Leave questions unanswered when your answer would be complete guesswork.
- Some MCQs are not negatively marked and for these you should answer all the questions, even if you have to guess.

Extended Matching Questions (EMQs)

Extended matching questions are increasingly being used for medical student exams. By using cases rather than just facts they can be used to test problem solving and the application of knowledge. Usually a clinical scenario (a vignette) is described and candidates are offered a list of up to 20 possible responses. The candidate has to select the single best answer for each vignette. Most commonly, several vignettes are grouped together within a clinical theme for a single set of responses. The best response may be used once, more than once or not at all, so don't be worried about this. Confusingly, it seems a common format is to list the responses before starting the vignettes. This type of question has the potential to be confusing so make sure you understand the format and practise answering such questions well in advance of the exam.

Short Answer Questions

The examiners will be awarding marks on the basis of individual points mentioned. Once again there will be few marks which can be flexibly awarded and no marks for points in the answer which do not address the question as actually asked. It is usually not necessary (or possible time-wise) to do a plan, but in many ways the answers should have the obvious structure of a plan. As with essay questions you should first of all spend a few minutes reading the instructions and all the questions twice. Then decide which questions you are going to answer and calculate the time to be spent on each question. Do not spend more time on any one question and make sure you finish all the questions.

It is important to deal with this part of the exam with care and a pre-pared approach. You should also aim to practise written answers before the exam. Except for clinical cases or OSCEs, marking is usually done anonymously by two examiners. Remember that many examiners attach great importance to legibility, accuracy and clearness of expression. In most universities answers have to be written into specific mark books and there are often requirements to write candidate numbers on each page, start each answer on a new sheet, etc. Try to follow these instructions in full. It may be advisable to use alternate lines in an answer book if this improves legibility, and it may also be a good idea to underline section headings, perhaps with a different colour. Use an appropriate pen for writ-ten answers and avoid unusual colours of ink. Resist the temptation to write so quickly that your writing becomes illegible.

Essay Questions

Many exams these days do not have essay questions. It would not harm you to practise writing essays, however, in preparation for any exam as they are a great way to sort your thoughts out in a logical manner. Writing an essay to a time limit is a definite skill which can be enormously improved with practice. It is obvious that one should read the questions carefully before starting to answer the paper, but it is amazing how many students apparently fail to do this.

The examiners will usually have decided in advance on an approxi-mate allocation of marks for each point made and discussed. There may be some spare marks to award arbitrarily for excellence but they will be relatively few. What this means is that you will get most of the marks for simply mentioning or sketching out points and relatively few for elaboration. If you spend time answering things which have not been asked, no matter how good your answer is, there will be no marks. An example would be where the examiner asks "How might a peptic ulcer present?" and the candidate spends time discussing how it might be treated.

Many medical schools (and postgraduate exams like the MRCS) use close marking schemes. The essence of these is that questions are all given marks close to the pass mark, i.e. 40 for a bad fail, 65 for a very good answer. This means that it is very difficult to make up for answers left completely unattempted. The only way to avoid simple types of error is to have a set plan of approach; since it is easy to make an error in the heat of battle, you must plan your strategy in advance. We would suggest the following.

SAMPLE QUESTIONS

Long Case Clerkings

Case 1

Mr. JS is a 67-year-old retired builder. He has attended today for the purpose of the exams. He presents with a year's history of progressive pain in his left hip. Over the last three months, however, the pain has worsened, and it now interferes with his sleep. He occasionally needs a stick and has particular difficulty in climbing stairs. Whereas in the past he could walk long distances, he can now only walk 200 yd before he is limited by pain in the groin and he also has difficulty in putting on his shoes and socks. His GP prescribed ibuprofen, which despite some initial help is now of no use.

There has been no history of trauma and he denies any problems with his other joints. He is married and lives in a two-storey house with his wife.

In his past medical history he had an appendicectomy at age 12 but otherwise has been fit and well, with no cardiorespiratory disease. He has no relevant family history and his only medication is ibuprofen. He denies any allergies and does not smoke or drink.

On systems review the only positive findings were those of prostatism, where he reports nocturia twice nightly, a poor stream and terminal dribbling of his urine.

On examination he is slightly overweight (weighing 110 kg, with a height of 5 ft 6 in). (If you can work out the body mass index (BMI), you certainly would impress the examiners. Note: BMI = weight^2 (kg)/height (cm) and is normally under 25.) But he looks generally well, with no signs of anaemia, jaundice or lymphadenopathy. Cardiorespiratory examination was unremarkable (have it written, in case the examiners ask you about any particular point), and abdominal examination revealed an appendicectomy scar. I did not perform a rectal examination but would normally do so, to feel the size and consistency of his prostate.

On examination of his hips he has an antalgic gait with a positive Trendelenburg's test. There is no leg length discrepancy. He has a fixed flexion deformity of 10° on the left side and a decreased range of movement of the left hip (flexion 10–85°, abduction 35°, adduction 10°, internal rotation 10° and external rotation 15°). The movements were most painful in full flexion and internal rotation. Examination of the right hip and the back and both knees was normal. There was no neurovascular deficit and no signs of peripheral vascular or venous disease.

In summary, this 67-year-old retired builder has a year's history of progressively worsening pain in his left hip which is now affecting his lifestyle and ability to sleep at night. My provisional diagnosis is that of osteoarthritis.

The examiners will then ask what investigations you would like to perform (plain X-rays) and will make you comment on them. They are likely to ask you about anything you have said.

If your diagnosis is correct, then the questions they may ask you are as follows:

- What is the treatment? (Conservative vs. surgical — lose weight, physio, etc., although the patient is likely to need a hip replacement.)
- You say in your history that he has prostatism — is that relevant? (Yes, he may go into postoperative retention.)
- The examiners may talk to the patient and ask you about your positive findings. (Trendelenburg's test, leg length, fixed flexion, Thomas's test.)

Case 2

Mrs. JP is a 51-year-old housewife who is currently an inpatient at this hospital, awaiting surgery. She presents with a lump in her left breast. She first noticed the lump two weeks ago whilst showering and it has not changed since then. She has no symptoms from the lump and she had never noticed any breast lumps before. Her main concern is that this is a cancer.

Her menarche was at age 12 and her periods were always regular up until her menopause two years ago. She has been on hormone replacement therapy since. She has no family history of breast cancer. She went to her GP, who sent her to the breast clinic last week, where she underwent a needle test and a mammography. She says the results were suggestive of cancer and she has been admitted for surgery. She has no relevant past medical history and is on no medication, but is allergic to penicillin, which gives her a rash. She lives with her husband John, who is 57, and they elected to have no children. She smokes ten cigarettes a day and drinks only occasionally.

Systems review was negative for any problems in the cardiovascular, respiratory, abdominal and neurological systems. On examination she looks well and is not pale or jaundiced. Examination of her breasts reveals that both nipples are inverted, although she says this has been present for as long as she can remember. She has a 3 cm hard lump in the upper outer quadrant of her left breast. The lump has an irregular outline but is mobile and not tethered to the chest wall or the skin. She has no lymphadenopathy and no evidence of metastatic spread on examination of her abdomen, chest and spine. Cardiorespiratory examination was unremarkable.

In summary, this 51-year-old postmenopausal lady has a suspicious 3 cm lump in her left breast. She has undergone triple assessment in the clinic and has been admitted for surgery tomorrow.

The examiners will ask questions like these:

- What is your differential diagnosis? (Benign or malignant cancer, fat necrosis, fibroadenoma (rare in this age group).)
- If you saw this lady in the clinic what investigations would you perform? (Triple assessment.)

- Are there any further investigations that can be performed? (Trucut and staging procedures.)
- What treatments are available?

Sample OSCE Station 1

"This patient has a lump in the left groin. Please examine it and say what you think it is."

(The station consists of a male patient with a left inguinal hernia, on a couch.)

Table 17.1 shows a possible marking scheme.

Sample OSCE Station 2

"Here is a 25-year-old man who presented at A&E with an 18 h history of acute abdominal pain. Please carry out an appropriate examination of his abdomen."

(The station consists of an actor in a gown and underpants, on a couch.)

Table 17.2 shows a possible marking scheme.

Table 17.1. Sample Marking Scheme

	Available marks = 10
Washes hands	0/1
Introduces themselves to patient and asks permission to examine them. Adequate exposure, preserves patient's dignity	0/1
Asks patient to point to site of lump	0/1
Stands patient up	0/1
Asks patient to cough and inspects for lump	0/1/2
Palpates anatomical landmarks	0/1/2
Defines position of lump in relation to testicle	0/1/2
Identifies it as an inguinal hernia	0/1

Table 17.2.   Sample Marking Scheme

	Available marks = 20
Introduces themselves and asks permission to examine patient	0/1/2
Washes hands	0/1/2
Arranges adequate exposure whilst preserving patient's dignity	0/1/2
Inspects abdomen	0/1/2
Palpates lightly all quadrants	0/1/2
Palpates deeply all quadrants	0/1/2
Feels for liver, spleen, kidneys	0/1/2
Examines hernial orifices	0/1/2
Percussion	0/1/2
Listens to bowel sounds	0/1/2

A wealth of sample MCQ questions and answers can be found in our sister textbook, which we recommend that you buy as a companion to this text.*

---

* Goldberg A. and Stansby G. (2008). *Surgery: Problems and Solutions. Revision Questions in Undergraduate Surgery (Clinical Talk Vol. 1)*. London: Imperial College Press. ISBN 9781848161870.